58

bbq

# Fundamentals of Abdominal Sonography

## A Teaching Approach

# Howard W. Raymond, M.D.

Radiologist and Chief of Ultrasound
Department of Radiology
Union-Truesdale Hospital
Fall River, Massachusetts

Clinical Instructor of Diagnostic Radiology
Brown University, Medical School
Providence, Rhode Island

 Grune & Stratton
*A Subsidiary of Harcourt Brace Jovanovich, Publishers*
New York     San Francisco     London

**Library of Congress Cataloging in Publication Data**

Raymond, Howard W
  Fundamentals of abdominal sonography.

  Bibliography
  Includes index.
    1. Abdomen—Diseases—Diagnosis.   2. Diagnosis,
Ultrasonic.   I. Title.
RC944.R29        617'.55'0754        78-26441
ISBN 0-8089-1144-9

*Grune & Stratton, Inc.*
*111 Fifth Avenue*
*New York, New York   10003*

Distributed in the United Kingdom by
*Academic Press, Inc. (London) Ltd.*
*24/28 Oval Road, London NW1*

Library of Congress Catalog Number 78-26441
International Standard Book Number 0-8089-1144-9

Printed in the United States of America

*This book is dedicated to my wife, Maxene, who helped me throughout all phases of the preparation of this book. I have sought her advice before making many important decisions; and in matters of judgment, although I may not always admit it, my wife is usually right.*

# Contents

# Acknowledgments

Writing a book such as this in a setting other than a teaching hospital requires the volunteer services of many individuals. The overall quality of the book relies in a large part on the quality of the illustrations. I would thus like to thank Jeanne Ferreira, whose assistance in the preparation of the illustrations was of immeasurable help to me.

My associates, Drs. Charles Mandell and Jagdish Shah, in addition to tolerating me while I was working on the book, offered valuable criticism in all phases of its preparation. I would also like to thank the members of the Department of Ultrasound, Josephine Houghton and David Charbonneau, for their expert work and pertinent suggestions.

I would like to acknowledge Rita O'Loughlin for her help in the typing of the manuscript. She aided me in such detailed and monotonous work as the preparation of the references, and somehow maintained her usual cheerful disposition throughout.

I would like, particularly, to thank the chief of the departments of Ultrasound and Nuclear Medicine, Herta Smith, for her assistance, not only in the preparation of this book, but for her help in developing the Department of Ultrasound. Without her dedication to excellence, this book would not have been possible.

Finally, I would like to thank my good friend Dr. Robert Knight, to whom I assigned the very important job of reading the manuscript. Criticism is sometimes difficult to take, but its bite is lessened when it is offered by a dear friend. I have no doubt that portions of this book are more intelligible because of Bob's recommendations.

# Preface

Radiologists in practice today are faced with a peculiar dilemma; they share with the clinician the pressures of improving bed utilization and holding down medical costs, and they are faced with a number of new diagnostic modalities at their disposal. Not only must they know how to interpret the various images presented to them, whether x-rays, scintigrams, sonograms, or computerized scans, but they must know how and where each study fits into the total diagnostic framework. If two diagnostic studies yield the same results, the radiologist may be criticized for duplication of effort which ultimately results in a longer hospital stay and increased costs. On the other hand, some duplication is necessary to provide the confidence level that clinicians have come to expect.

The literature in one of these new modalities, ultrasound, abounds with controversy over the indications for various procedures. Obviously there are times when sonography is useful and times when it is not; but the field is new, and universal agreement over specific indications has not been established. As a general radiologist in a moderate-sized community hospital, I generally get involved with the entire imaging workup, including x-ray, nuclear medicine, and ultrasound, and I do feel the pressure from clinicians to use the means at my disposal in a most efficient manner. In many instances I have found a particular sonographic study to provide information where other modalities fail, while in other areas I have been disappointed with its value. I have tried to indicate these conclusions within this book.

Another dilemma faced by the modern radiologist is how to interpret these new images, for the perspective is different from that of the conventional x-ray: instead of frontal, lateral, and oblique projections, sonograms represent thin sagittal and transverse sections. Moreover, the scans appear foreign because the interaction of sound within the body is different than x-radiation. One must, therefore, learn a new series of fundamental principles and signs.

This book is also directed to the ultrasound technologist, who is, of course, responsible for performing a thorough examination and obtaining readable scans. Unlike technologists in other imaging modalities, ultrasound technologists must have a workable knowledge of abdominal anatomy and pathology. The quality of their work will ultimately depend not only on their technical ability, but on their understanding of the normal and abnormal images viewed on the monitor. The dialogue between the ultrasound technologist and physician is, and I believe will continue to remain, a very essential element of the sonographic examination.

This book is an attempt to describe an approach, first, to the utilization of ultrasound in the overall diagnostic workup and, second, to the interpretation of the scans. To achieve this end, I have taken a few lessons from my former chief, Dr. Benjamin Felson, in constructing a teaching format for the field of abdominal ultrasound. The reader is advised to examine each case as it is presented and to make conclusions before proceeding to the discussion of the case. The reader is put "on the spot" to make his or her own diagnosis. This format will, I hope, stimulate thought and make the subject matter more absorbing.

# 1

# Abdominal Sonogram

A basic abdominal sonographic study with the systematic collection of transverse and sagittal scans should serve as the groundwork for any abdominal sonogram. Because of the posterior location of the kidneys, of course, renal echography demands an entirely different sonic approach that will be discussed in Chapter 6. The gallbladder, pancreatic, liver, and aortic studies performed in our department, however, are modifications of the basic abdominal sonogram. The particular modifications that enable us to better examine the organ under question will be discussed at the beginning of the respective chapters.

No doubt there are as many techniques for this study as there are institutions that perform it. Outlined below is the abdominal examination performed at our institution. In the scans shown, the important organs and vascular structures are pointed out.

In keeping with the prevailing convention, all sagittal scans are shown so that the patients head (H) is on the reader's left as he or she views the scan. All transverse scans are shown with the patient's right side on the reader's left, similar to the manner in which AP roentgenograms are viewed. The patient's right side will be denoted by the letter *R*. Because of the instrumentation, the right and left sides are reversed in the prone transverse scans. For example, the right kidney will be on the reader's right, while the left kidney will be on the reader's left. To avoid confusion, both *R* and *L* will be used on the scans. Oblique, decubitus, and other scans that do not lie in the sagittal or transverse planes will be appropriately labeled.

Nearly all the longitudinal scans were obtained in the semidecubitus position described in Chapter 2 (p. 18). In the figure legends, the position of the patient will be specified only if it is other than semidecubitus. Similarly, it is to be assumed that all transverse scans were obtained in the supine position, unless otherwise stated.

Black and white background scans are used in this book; occasionally, both backgrounds are used in the same case, and in a few cases the same scan is reproduced with both backgrounds. We have found that each type of scan offers

1

advantages and, therefore, use them interchangeably. Most of our recent work, however, is with white background.

We begin with supine transverse scans beginning just below the xyphoid and proceed caudally at 1-cm. intervals until the liver and right kidney are no longer visualized. The transducer arm is placed in the midline remaining stationary, while the angle of the transducer, with respect to the patient, is changed. In a manner of speaking, the transducer is rotated from right to left or vice versa (Figs. 1-1A, 1-1B, 1-2A, 1-2B, 1-3A, 1-3B).

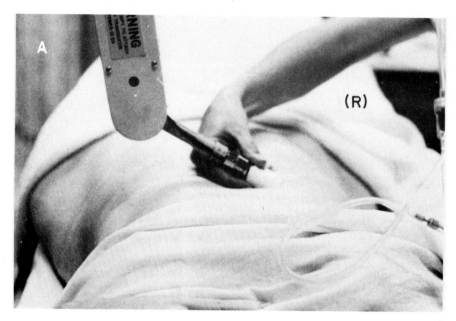

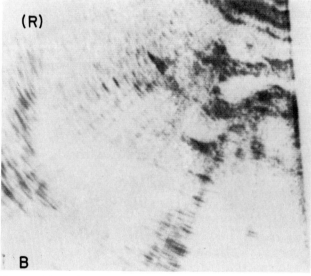

**Fig. 1-1.**   (A) The transducer is angled to the right. (B) Limited sector scan with transducer angled to the right.

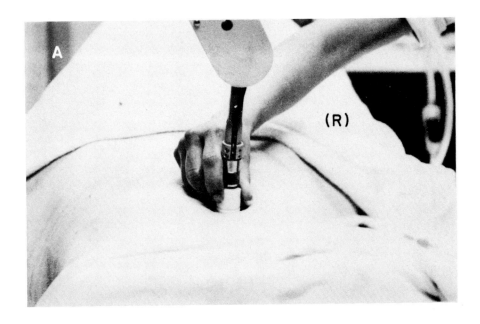

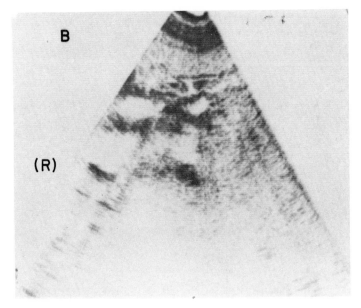

**Fig. 1-2.** (A) The transducer is directed perpendicular to the epigastrium. (B) Limited sector scan of epigastrium.

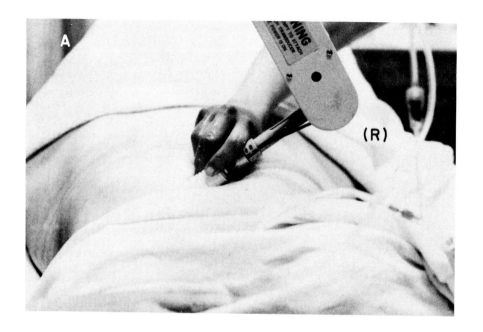

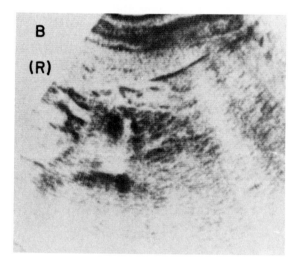

**Fig. 1-3.** (A) The transducer is angled to the left. (B) Limited sector scan with transducer angled to the left.

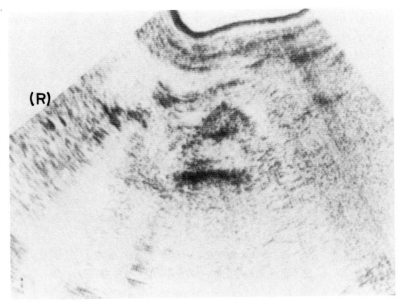

**Fig. 1-4.** "Pie" scan of the epigastrium.

As a result, pie scans of approximately 120 degrees, depending on the patient, are obtained (Fig. 1-4).*

This is a very essential technique for proper scans. Maximal resolution is desirable, indeed necessary, for evaluation of the vessels in the epigastrium. By passing the sound beam over the area of interest as quickly as the writing speed of the instrument permits, one minimizes the effects of respiration and other movements. Another way of attaining maximal resolution is to use the highest frequency transducer that will allow adequate penetration. Whenever possible, we use the 3.5 MHz transducer with either a 7.5 or 10cm focus, depending on the patient's body structure.

Many such sector scans may be performed until the technologist feels that an optimal picture is obtained, which is one of the reasons it is imperative for a technologist to know abdominal and vascular anatomy. After an optimal sector scan is obtained, the remainder of the picture is filled in by compound scanning around the lower thorax and upper abdomen from costovertebral angle to costovertebral angle, being careful not to sector through the epigastrium again (Fig. 1-5).

This technique poses a problem of manual dexterity with many of the sector scanners, but can generally be overcome by experience. A good scan should contain exquisitely detailed information in the epigastrium and adequate detail laterally to evaluate the kidneys, spleen, liver, and gallbladder. Aside from technical skill, other factors such as gas and obesity limit the quality of the transverse

*All studies in this book, with the exceptions of Fig. 5-16, 5-18, and 5-28, were performed with a Picker Corp. Echoview 80L System.

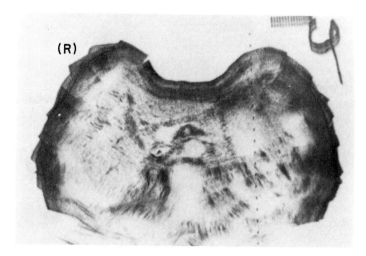

**Fig. 1-5.** Completed transverse scan.


scans. In our experience, an adequate study can be obtained in approximately 80 percent of patients.

A typical examination is shown in the following figures. Of course, because of patient variability, the particular structures may be encountered at different levels. At the xyphoid (Fig. 1-6), the aorta (Ao) and inferior vena cava (IVC) are seen. The liver (L) fills most of the right side of the abdomen. On the left, gas in the stomach (arrows) obliterates much of the anatomy. The shadow cast by the spine (S) is noted posteriorly.

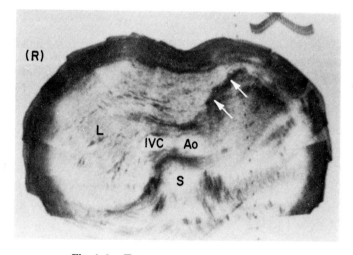

**Fig. 1-6.** Transverse scan at the xyphoid.

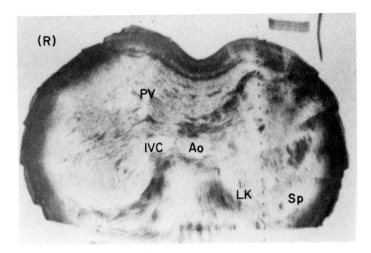

**Fig. 1-7.** Transverse scan at the xyphoid −1 cm.

At 1 cm below the xyphoid (Fig. 1-7), branches of the portal vein (PV) are seen within the liver. The spleen (Sp) can be seen posteriolaterally and the top of the left kidney is identified (LK).

At 2 cm below the xyphoid (Fig.1-8), we can begin to appreciate the main portal vein (MPV). The pelvocalyceal clump of echoes within the left kidney is noted (arrow).

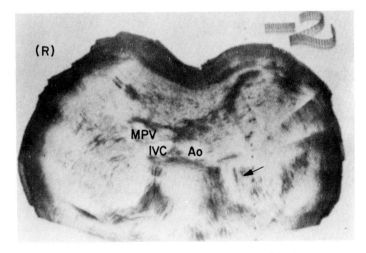

**Fig. 1-8.** Transverse scan at the xyphoid −2 cm.

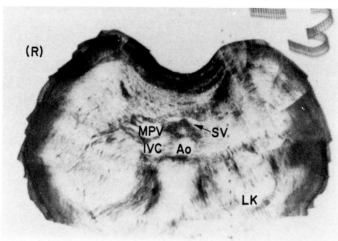

**Fig. 1-9.**   Transverse scan at the xyphoid −3 cm.

At 3 cm below the xyphoid (Fig. 1-9), the main portal vein (MPV) is clearly seen and the splenic vein (SV) begins to come into view.

At 4 cm below the xyphoid (Fig. 1-10), one can appreciate the confluence of the splenic and superior mesenteric veins to form the portal vein (PV). The superior mesenteric artery (SMA) is identified anterior to the aorta and posterior to the splenic vein. A vessel is seen passing to the IVC from the left between the SMA and aorta. This is the left renal vein (LRV).

A limited sector scan at this level (Fig. 1-11A, 1-11B) will reveal the head and neck of the pancreas (outlined in Fig. 1-11B). The pancreatic tissue (P) is somewhat more echogenic than the adjacent liver (L).

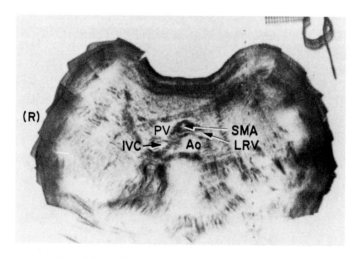

**Fig. 1-10.**   Transverse scan at the xyphoid −4 cm.

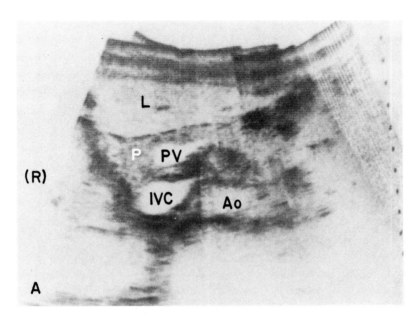

**Fig. 1-11A.** Transverse sector scan at the xyphoid −4 cm.

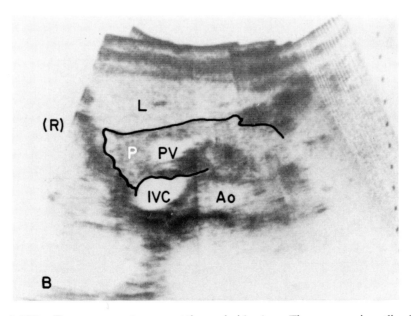

**Fig. 1-11B.** Transverse sector scan at the xyphoid −4 cm. The pancreas is outlined.

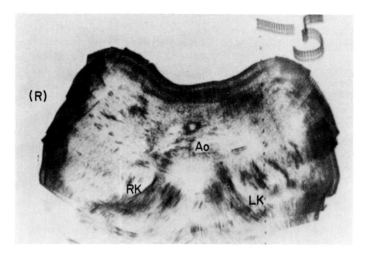

**Fig. 1-12.**   Transverse scan at the xyphoid −5 cm.

At 5 cm below the xyphoid (Fig. 1-12), the top of the right kidney (RK) comes into view. Though not the case with this patient, the gallbladder is frequently seen at this level.

At 6 cm below the xyphoid (Fig. 1-13), one can identify the gallbladder, which is small in this particular patient. The right kidney (RK) is well seen. Gas obscures much of the left side of the abdomen. Further 1 cm sections are taken until gas obliterates the structures within the abdomen. Our technicians do scan the entire abdomen searching for lower abdominal aortic aneurysms, large masses, ab-

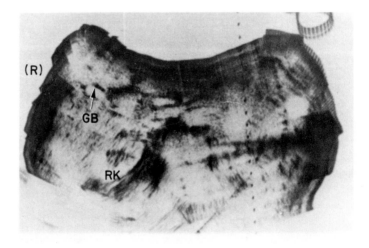

**Fig. 1-13.**   Transverse scan at the xyphoid −6 cm.

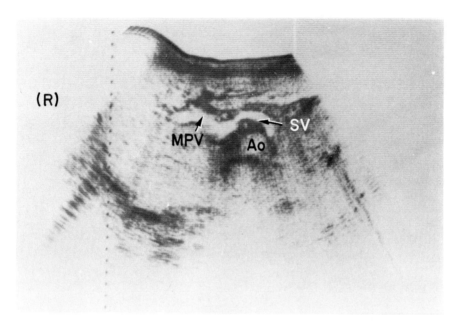

**Fig. 1-14.**   Transverse scan showing splenic vein (SV) and main portal vein (MPV).

scesses, and other pathology. If such conditions are present, of course, representative pictures are taken.

The relationship between the splenic and portal veins may be appreciated on the transverse section (Fig. 1-14). The splenic vein (SV) crosses over the SMA and joins the superior mesenteric vein (SMV) to become the main portal vein (MPV). The MPV passes toward the hilum of the liver and divides into right and left branches.

In thin patients, one may identify the right renal artery (RA) (Fig. 1-15A,) and celiac axis (CA) (Fig. 1-15B), by using a high frequency transducer.

The longitudinal scans begin at the midline or over the aorta and proceed to the right at 1 cm intervals until the shape of the thorax prevents further scanning. A combination technique is used to obtain these longitudinal scans. The sweep begins with a sector scan that moves from a cranial-most direction, which is usually the right hemidiaphragm, and ends with the transducer surface perpendicular to the patient. The remainder of the anatomy is filled in by simply sliding the transducer in a longitudinal direction over the surface of the patient, keeping the contact surface perpendicular to the abdomen. This completion of the picture may give important information about the right kidney, aorta, inferior vena cava, and pancreas, but is often obscured by gas.

At the midline or just to the left of the midline (Fig. 1-16), the aorta (Ao) is well seen. The celiac axis (CA), the first recognizable branch of the abdominal aorta, may occasionally be identified. Just below the celiac axis, the superior mesenteric artery (SMA) arises and passes anterior to the aorta.

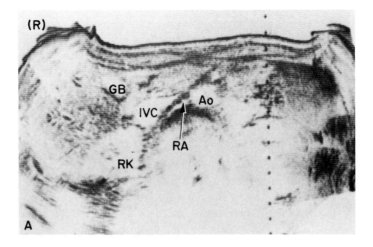

**Fig. 1-15A.** Transverse scan showing right renal artery (RA).

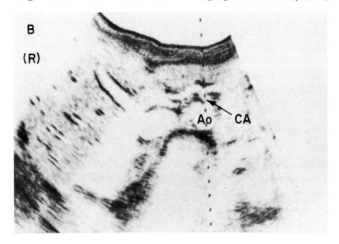

**Fig. 1-15B.** Transverse scan showing celiac axis (CA).

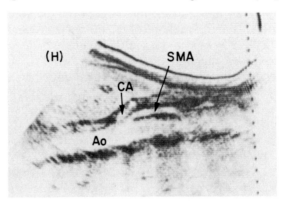

**Fig. 1-16.** Longitudinal scan showing aorta (Ao), celiac axis (CA) and superior mesenteric artery (SMA).

The superior mesenteric vein (SMV) (Fig. 1-17A, 1-17B) is anterior to the superior mesenteric artery (SMA) and is generally a larger and more sonolucent vessel than the SMA. The SMV lies either in the same sagittal plane or just to the right of the aorta. The SMV is particularly important to identify because of its relationship to the neck of the pancreas (P).

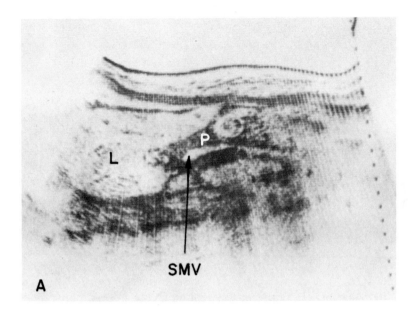

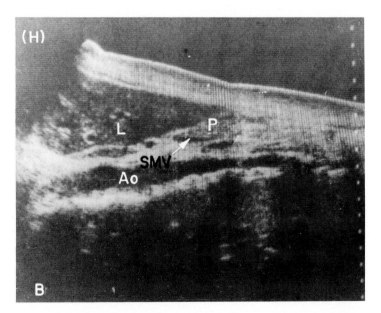

**Fig. 1-17.** (A) Longitudinal scan showing relationship of superior mesenteric vein (SMV) to the pancreas (P), on white background. (B) Similar scan, on black background.

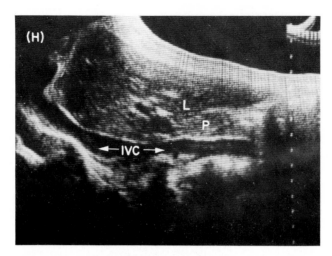

**Fig. 1-18.** Longitudinal scan of inferior vena cava (IVC).

The inferior vena cava (IVC) (Fig. 1-18,) lies somewhat to the right of the aorta and is also an important structure to identify because of its relationship to the pancreatic head (P). This structure has a very variable size, shape, and position in both the longitudinal and transverse sections.

As one proceeds further toward the right (Fig. 1-19), one will encounter the gallbladder (GB). The cross section of the right portal vein (RPV) is frequently seen in the same plane. With careful scanning, the normal common bile duct (CBD) may be identified.

Finally, the right kidney (RK) may be scanned through the right lobe of the

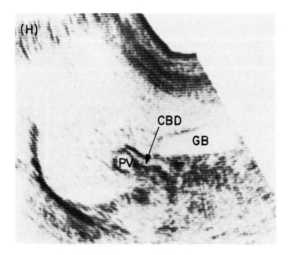

**Fig. 1-19.** Longitudinal scan showing right portal vein (RPV), common bile duct (CBD), and gallbladder (GB).

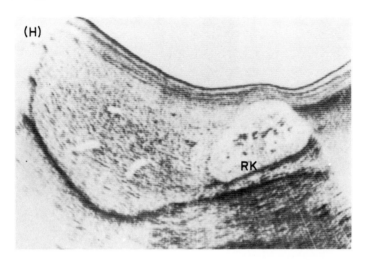

(H)

RK

**Fig. 1-20.** Longitudinal scan showing right kidney (RK).

liver (Fig. 1-20). Frequently this scan provides the best view of the right kidney. Gas in the right upper quadrant may obscure the lower pole, but with a certain degree of skill the technician may be able to get around the gas and visualize the entire right kidney. A myriad of other vessels and structures in the upper abdomen can be visualized, but this has little practical value in the diagnosis of disease. We have found the basic examination described above sufficient as a foundation for the biliary system, pancreas, and liver studies. Because of the location of the kidneys, a completely different approach is required and will be discussed in Chapter 6.

## SUGGESTED READINGS

Albarelli JN, Hagan SL, McKay L, et al: Gray scale sonographic atlas of anatomy and pathology. Picker Corporation, 1976, pp 93–108

Carlsen EN, Filly RA: Newer ultrasonographic anatomy in the upper abdomen: I. The portal and hepatic venous anatomy. J Clin Ultrasound 4:85–91, 1976

Filly RA, Carlsen EN: Newer ultrasonographic anatomy in the upper abdomen: II. The major systemic veins and arteries with a special note on localization of the pancreas. J Clin Ultrasound 4:91–96, 1976

Garrett WJ, Kosseff G, Carpenter DA: Gray scale compound scan echography of the normal upper abdomen. J Clin Ultrasound 3:199–204, 1975

Sample WF: Techniques for improved delineation of normal anatomy of the upper abdomen and high retroperitoneum with gray-scale ultrasound. Radiology 124:197–202, 1977

Weill F, Eisenscher A, Aucant A, et al: Ultrasonic study of the venous patterns in the hypochondrium: An anatomical approach to differential diagnosis. J Clin Ultrasound 3:23–28, 1975

# 2
# Gallstones

In the past three years, gallbladder sonography has become a routine diagnostic procedure. Accuracy rates reported in the recent literature are between 72 and 100 percent, with most falling at around 90 percent.[1-6] Aside from its obvious value in the detection of gallstones, ultrasonic evaluation of the upper abdomen may reveal many other associated and nonassociated conditions. Indeed, much of the pathology presented in this book was discovered during routine gallbladder sonography. Ultrasound may eventually come to be used as a screening procedure in the abdomen.

## INDICATIONS

As with any new procedure, the indications for sonographic cholecystography are controversial. Some authors have recently suggested using gallbladder sonography as the initial screening procedure in patients suspected of having acute or chronic biliary tract disease.[7] Others have taken a more moderate stance and have listed specific situations where this modality is useful.[8] Our experience has led us to conclusions very similar to those reported by the latter authors.

At our institution, we perform this study on the following category of patients: (1) those with elevated serum bilirubin levels in whom an oral cholecystogram would not be possible: (2) those with nonvisualized gallbladders after a single oral dose (We still use the oral cholecystogram as the initial screening procedure when possible): (3) those with symptoms of acute cholecystitis: and (4) those in whom, for various reasons, adequate spot filming of the gallbladder cannot or should not be performed, for example, obese or pregnant patients.

Many clinicians at our institution now prefer to order gallbladder sonography rather than oral cholecystography on their patients. The side effects of oral contrast, although certainly not dangerous, are often uncomfortable and inconvenient. The accuracy rate of ultrasound cholecystography at the present time is approximately 90 percent and will probably approach 100 percent as the equip-

ment is perfected. At that time we should reconsider the use of the oral cholecystogram as the initial screening procedure.


## TECHNIQUE

The type of gallbladder sonogram performed in our department involves
more than just views of the gallbladder. We have found it useful to visualize other
organs in the upper abdomen, such as the liver, pancreas, kidneys, and aorta, and
have been impressed with the frequency with which related and incidental pathology have been discovered. It should be remembered that patients are often referred to the x-ray department for vague complaints which may be related to a
gamut of conditions. A typical example is a pancreatic pseudocyst discovered as
an incidental finding during a gallbladder examination. This is a sufficiently common experience to warrant a broader approach to the upper abdomen than the
mere visualization of the gallbladder.

The gallbladder sonogram performed in our department is a modification of
the basic abdominal study. The full complement of transverse and longitudinal
supine scans described in Chapter 1 are obtained, as well as several limited
longitudinal sector scans of the gallbladder. In addition to the basic longitudinal
scans, many sweeps are made of the gallbladder from its neck to the tip of the
fundus. If the gallbladder can be consistently seen during both inspiration and
expiration, no attempt is made to have the patient suspend respiration for all the
images obtained since, because of the number of passes taken to evaluate the
gallbladder, suspended respiration can become very tiresome for the patient. If
the gallbladder can be seen only during inspiration the patient must inhale deeply
while these limited sweeps are performed. The technologist takes three or four
pictures of what he or she considers representative scans (Fig. 2-1). If there are
ambiguous findings, several more pictures are taken.

Roughly 20 percent of gallbladders cannot be visualized by this technique.

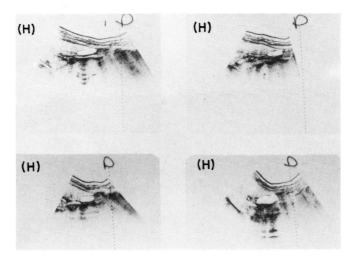

**Fig. 2-1.**   Longitudinal, limited sector scans of the gallbladder.

Five percent of these are in patients with livers placed high in the thorax. The gallbladder lies beneath the ribs in these patients even during maximal inspiration; in particular, stocky young men fit into this category. A limited examination can be performed on these patients by sectoring in the intercostal space close to the gallbladder. If gallstones are present, they may be visualized in this manner, but the examination is not sufficient to prove their absence. In the remaining 15 percent of the cases, gas obscures adequate visualization of the gallbladder. The gas generally will lie behind the gallbladder, making visualization of the acoustic shadow, if any, difficult.

To overcome this problem, the patient assumes a semidecubitus position by rolling on the left side approximately 30 degrees. The scanning arm is also angled 30 degrees (Fig. 2-2), and longitudinal scans of the right upper quadrant are obtained in much the same manner as the longitudinal, supine scans described in Chapter 1. Bowel loops that may have obscured the gallbladder in the supine position tend to fall toward the left, allowing better visualization of the gallbladder and stones if present. In this position, the right lobe of the liver will serve as an ideal window to visualize the gallbladder (Fig. 2-3). Moreover, other structures in

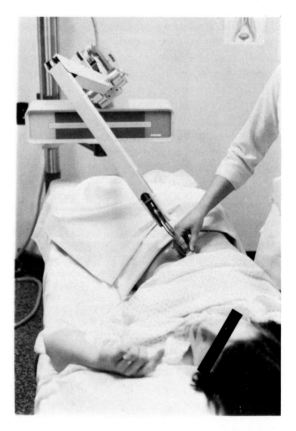

**Fig. 2-2.** Technique of semidecubitus longitudinal scan.
Note position of scanning arm and patient.

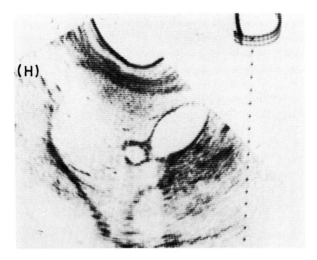

**Fig. 2-3.**  Typical semidecubitus longitudinal scan.

the upper abdomen, such as the inferior vena cava, right kidney, and common bile duct may be better visualized,

Occasionally, upright, longitudinal views of the gallbladder have been found to be useful (Fig. 2-4), but, as a practical matter, these scans can be obtained only in relatively thin patients. In general, the semidecubitus position has been found to be more practical for demonstrating changes in the position of stones. The upright scan is used only in questionable cases.

This complete examination may take anywhere between 20 and 30 minutes to perform. When completed, information about the gallbladder in several different planes and positions is obtained. Evaluation of the gallbladder alone would take a fraction of the time and effort. However, useful information about the liver,

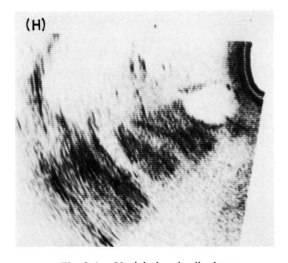

**Fig. 2-4.**  Upright longitudinal scan.

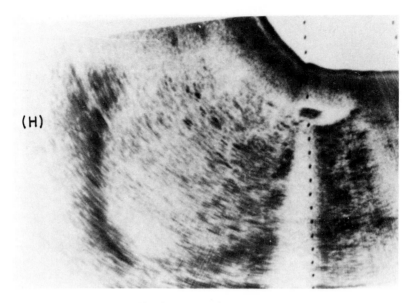

**Fig. 2-5.** Longitudinal scan.

kidneys, inferior vena cava, aorta, and pancreas is made available to the physician interpreting the study, and the additional time spent in performance of the complete study yields dividends well worth the effort.

## GALLSTONES

The classic stone (Fig. 2-5, 2-6) fulfills three criteria. It is (1) a discrete, echogenic density, (2) within a fluid-filled, sonolucent gallbladder, and (3) causes acoustic shadowing. Incidentally, can you identify other significant pathology in Figure 2-5?

The first criterion is self-evident. Diligent scanning in search of stones is

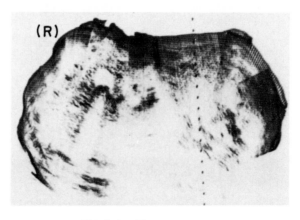

**Fig. 2-6.** Transverse scan.

particularly important when using a sector scanner. As demonstrated in Fig. 2-7A, 2-7B, a gallstone may be minute, as compared to the gallbladder lumen, and many sector scans may be necessary to delineate the stone and its shadow (arrows). Both white and black background scans are reproduced for comparison; however, it is generally easier to identify the acoustic shadow with black background.

Although the second criterion also seems self-evident, the fact is that the most difficult gallbladder to evaluate is the one filled with stones and little fluid. This problem will be considered in more detail later.

Finally, there has been considerable controversy concerning the third criterion, acoustic shadowing. As we have gained experience, we have found that the percentage of stones that do not shadow has declined. It is, therefore, likely that the failure to find shadows in the past was, in part, a function of technique. There is no doubt, however, that there are stones that do not shadow. Goldberg claims

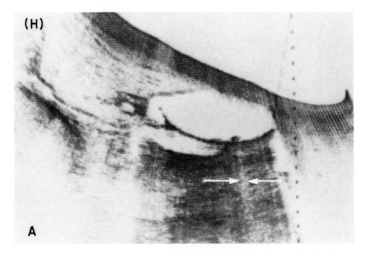

**Fig. 2-7A.**   Longitudinal scan. White background. Note acoustic shadow (arrows).

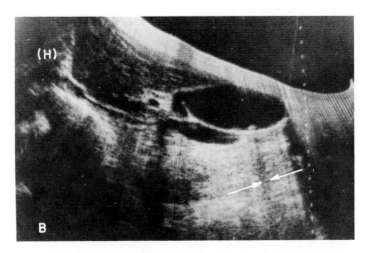

**Fig. 2-7B.**   Longitudinal scan. Black background. Note acoustic shadow (arrows).

that stones of high cholesterol and low calcium content tend to present without shadows.[9] In our experience, however, these are sufficiently rare to raise the suspicion of other disease entities, such as carcinoma of the gallbladder.

One must be less than definite when diagnosing a stone that does not shadow. Occasionally, a bowel loop will indent the flexible gallbladder and result in an appearance similar to a non-shadowing stone. Furthermore, a septated gallbladder may appear not unlike a nonshadowing stone (Fig. 2-8A, 2-8B).

Another problem presented by nonshadowing, echogenic material within the

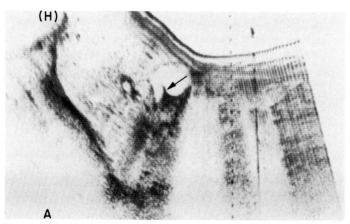

**Fig. 2-8A.**   Longitudinal scan. Note septation (arrow) within lumen of gallbladder.

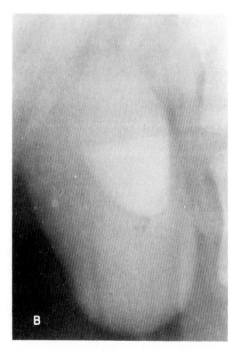

**Fig. 2-8B.**   Spot film of gallbladder.

gallbladder is sludge. Sludge may be found within normal gallbladders and should be differentiated from the pathological entity of gallstones. Some authors have advocated scanning the gallbladder in multiple positions—supine, erect, and decubitus.[10] Presumably, sludge, being very viscous, will settle into the dependent portion of the gallbladder very slowly, as compared to stones that fall as rapidly as the patient is moved.

Aside from stones, there may be other sonographic evidence to suggest inflammatory disease of the gallbladder. The walls of the normal gallbladder present a pencil-thin acoustic interface with the surrounding structures (Fig. 2-9A). Occasionally, the gallbladder walls become so thickened as a result of chronic inflammation that the acoustic interface widens enough to be appreciated on the scan (Fig. 2-9B). The diagnosis of chronic cholecystitis is suggested in cases such as these.

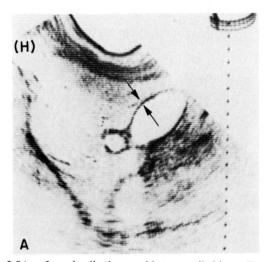

**Fig. 2-9A.**  Longitudinal scan. Note pencil-thin walls of the normal gallbladder (arrows).

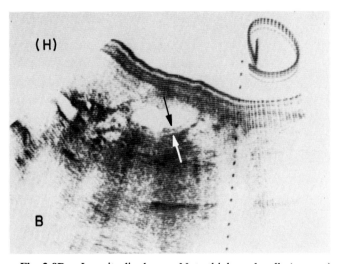

**Fig. 2-9B.**  Longitudinal scan. Note thickened walls (arrows).

**Case**

The scans shown in Figs. 2-10, 2-11 are longitudinal, semidecubitus and supine transverse views in a patient with a nonvisualizing gallbladder on oral cholecystography. What conclusions would you reach if you were presented with these scans?

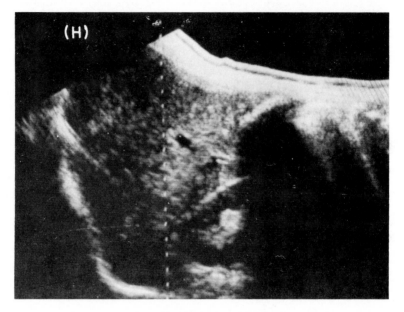

**Fig. 2-10.**   Longitudinal scan.

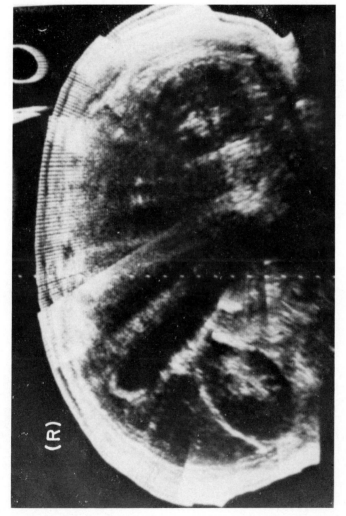

**Fig. 2-11.** Transverse scan.

DISCUSSION

It is tempting to throw up one's hands in despair and blame the problem on gas. There is no doubt that gas may obscure the gallbladder and on occasion may simulate gallstones. The semidecubitus position, however, alleviates this problem significantly. One may even be able to trace the shadow to the transverse colon which has a characteristic sonographic appearance (Fig. 2-12). Note the shadowing that is produced by the small amount of gas in this portion of the colon (arrows).

Another cause of shadowing in the right upper quadrant is calcification within the liver parenchyma (Fig. 2-13A, 2-13B).

A third cause of shadowing in the right upper quadrant is the gallbladder filled with stones. This problem has been alluded to in the first section of this chapter. Gallstone criteria are: (1) discrete, echogenic densities, (2) within a sonolucent gallbladder, and (3) causes acoustic shadowing. Although the second criterion, at first glance, appears to be self-evident, the so-called packed-bag is one of the most difficult gallbladders to evaluate. The case presented above is an example of a

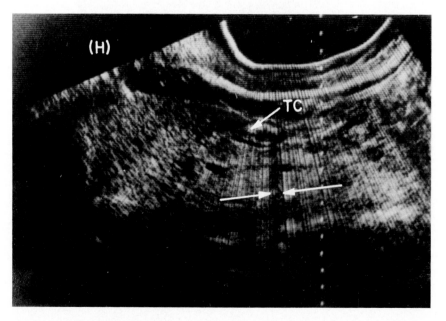

**Fig. 2-12.** Longitudinal scan. Note characteristic appearance of transverse colon (TC). There is a subtle acoustic shadow (arrows) caused by the gas in the colon.

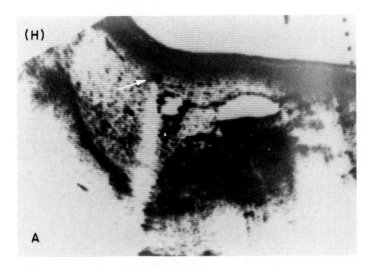

**Fig. 2-13A.** Longitudinal scan. Calcification within the liver parenchyma (arrow) causing acoustic shadowing.

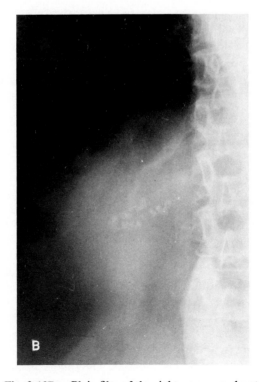

**Fig. 2-13B.** Plain film of the right upper quadrant.

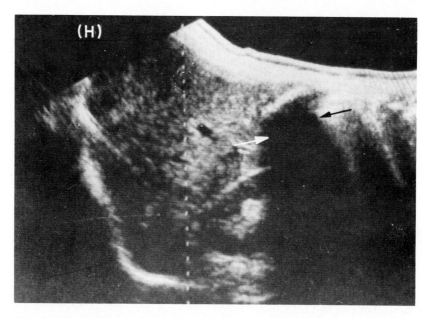

**Fig. 2-14.** Longitudinal scan. Note linear configuration of echogenic densities and sharp acoustic shadow (arrows).

packed gallbladder. In general, this condition may be suspected when the densities causing the shadows are discrete and very echogenic (Fig. 2-14). The shadowing that these densities produce is very sharply defined (arrows). Frequently, the densities themselves are aligned in a very straight horizontal fashion. This sonographic appearance remains constant in both the supine and semidecubitus positions. Anything resembling a normal gallbladder, of course, cannot be found.

FOLLOW UP

The patient went to surgery, and a gallbladder filled with stones was found.

COMMENTS

Despite the sonographic findings described, the diagnosis of a packed gallbladder must be made with some hesitancy. Further evaluation, including a KUB, or plain film of the abdomen (the stones may be calcified), oral cholecystogram, and even an intravenous cholangiogram, may be necessary.

In addition to the three causes of shadowing in the right upper quadrant (gas, liver calcification, and stones) described above, there is another less common condition which may result in a similar sonographic appearance. Fig. 2-15 is an example of this condition—calcification within the wall of the gallbladder, or porcelain gallbladder. This case resembles the packed gallbladder presented above. As one would expect, the echogenic density that represents the wall of the gallbladder tends to lie in a more crescentic fashion (arrows). This is not a very reliable sign, and a KUB should be obtained when there is doubt. The porcelain gallbladder, of course, has a characteristic x-ray appearance (Fig. 2-16).

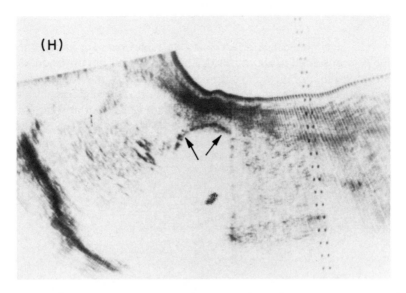

(H)

**Fig. 2-15.** Longitudinal scan. Note curvilinear configuration of echogenic density (arrows). Compare to Fig. 2-14.

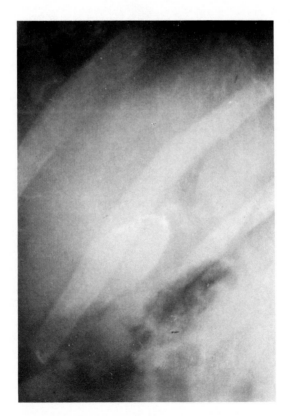

**Fig. 2-16.** Plain film of the right upper quadrant showing porcelain gallbladder.

## Case

LB is a 35-year-old female referred to our department for gallbladder sonography. She had presented to another hospital because of right upper quadrant pain and jaundice. Because of elevated serum bilirubin levels, more conventional studies, such as oral cholecystography and intravenous cholangiography, were not performed. Below are representative longitudinal (2 cm to the right of midline) and transverse scans (Fig. 2-17, 2-18). This case is presented mainly to demonstrate the anatomy. Can you name the numbered structures?

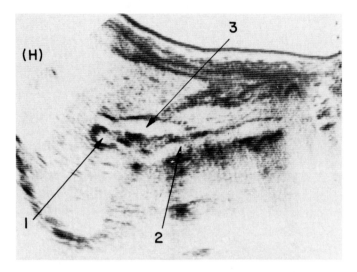

**Fig. 2-17.**   Longitudinal scan, 2 cm to right of midline.

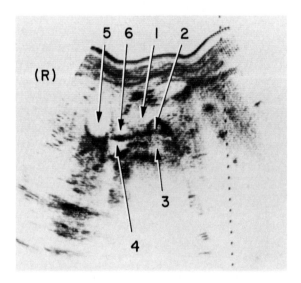

**Fig. 2-18.**   Transverse scan of epigastrium.

DISCUSSION

This patient had a dilated common bile duct due to an obstructing stone near the ampulla of Vater. In this case and others that follow, no distinction is made between the common bile and hepatic ducts. The longitudinal section (Fig. 2-19) reveals: (1) the portal vein, (2) the inferior vena cava, and (3) the common bile duct. In the longitudinal section, as the common bile duct is followed cranio-caudally, it passes over the portal vein and dips posterior to the pancreas and anterior to the inferior vena cava. Optimal visualization of the common bile duct is obtained in a semidecubitus position. The patient should, in addition, be slightly oblique so that the transducer passes from right to left as it sweeps caudally.

With careful scanning, a normal common bile duct may be identified. Fig. 2-20 is such a case. Again, the common bile duct (arrow) passes over the portal vein (PV) and behind the gallbladder (GB).

The transverse scan (Fig. 2-21) reveals: (1) the pancreas, (2) the superior mesenteric artery, (3) the aorta, (4) the inferior vena cava, (5) the gallbladder, and (6) the common bile duct. As demonstrated, the common bile duct lies medial to the gallbladder, anterior to the inferior vena cava, and adjacent to the pancreatic head. In general, a common duct of normal caliber has not been identified on transverse scans.

COMMENTS

1. This abnormal case has been presented because it demonstrates the anatomic relation of the common bile duct to other structures in the right upper quadrant. Visualization of a dilated common bile duct in both sagittal and trans-

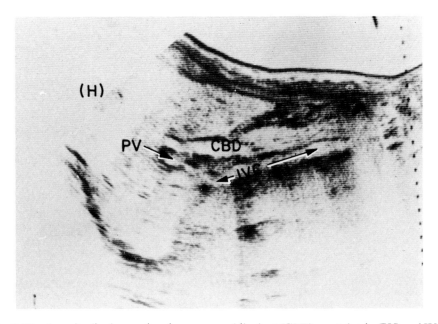

**Fig. 2-19.** Longitudinal scan showing common bile duct (CBD), portal vein (PV) and IVC.

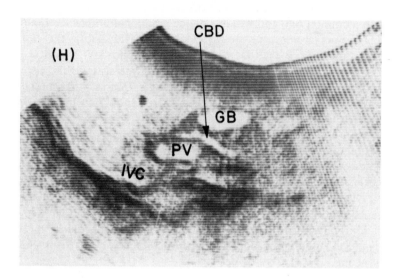

**Fig. 2-20.** Longitudinal scan in normal patient. Note position of CBD relative to the gallbladder (GB) and portal vein (PV).

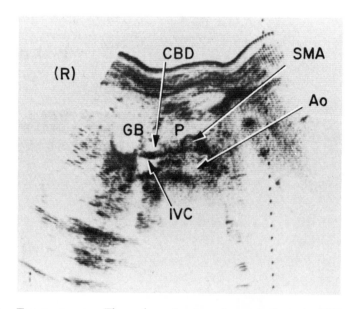

**Fig. 2-21.** Transverse scan. The various structures in proximity to the CBD are labeled.

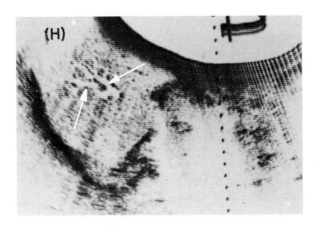

**Fig. 2-22.** Longitudinal scan. Note stellate configuration of dilated biliary ducts (arrows).

verse planes has frequently been possible. It should be mentioned, however, that this structure, even when dilated, may be difficult to visualize in certain patients.

2. Because of the relatively acute nature of the problem, this patient did not have dramatic enlargement of the small intrahepatic biliary ducts. Above are longitudinal scans of the liver in a patient with dilated intrahepatic bile ducts (Fig. 2-22). A normal longitudinal scan of the liver is reproduced for comparison (Fig. 2-23). Centrally, the dilated bile ducts assume a stellate pattern described by Taylor, as they emanate from the *porta hepatis* (Fig. 2-22, arrows).[11] The hepatic veins, on the other hand, are generally seen in long, straight channels without recognizable walls (Fig. 2-23, arrows).

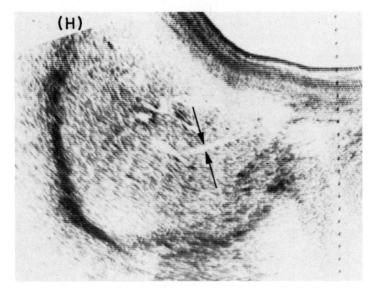

**Fig. 2-23.** Longitudinal scan. Arrows point at hepatic vein.

3.  It may be difficult to differentiate between dilated branches of the portal vein and bile ducts. In general, on the sagittal section, the small portal branches are viewed in cross section as compared to the bile ducts which are seen in a more longitudinal orientation. Conrad and associates have reported the parallel channel sign which is useful in identifying subtle distention of the biliary tree.[12] This particular sign will be discussed in more detail in the next chapter.
4.  Real time imaging is a helpful improvement for studying the various vessels within the liver. With real time systems, one is able to trace the various channels to their origins. For example, the hepatic veins can easily be traced into the inferior vena cava, the small portal branches may be traced into the main portal vein, and the biliary radicles, if dilated, may be traced into the common hepatic or common bile ducts.

### Case

OR is a 23-year-old female with right upper quadrant pain. Longitudinal and transverse sonograms of the right upper quadrant are reproduced below (Fig.2-24, 2-25). What conclusions can you make about these scans in addition to the gallstones?

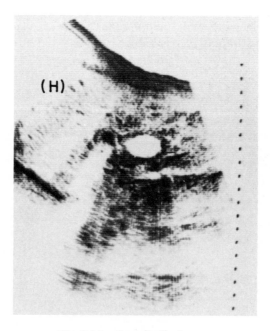

**Fig. 2-24.**   Longitudinal scan.

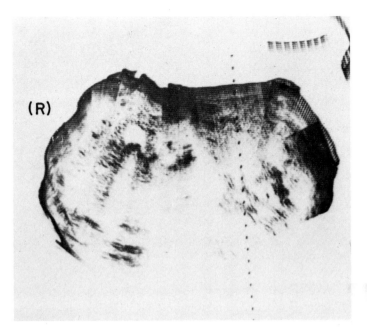

**Fig. 2-25.** Transverse scan.

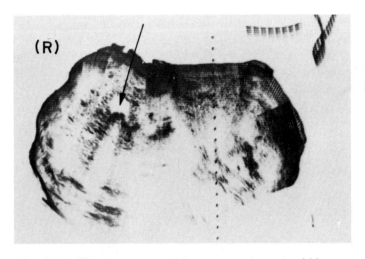

**Fig. 2-26.** Transverse scan. Note stones (arrow) within gallbladder.

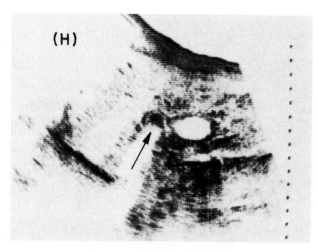

**Fig. 2-27.**   Longitudinal scan.  Note stone at neck of gallbladder (arrow).

DISCUSSION

The transverse scan reveals the presence of classic stones within the lumen
of the gallbladder (Fig. 2-26). The longitudinal scan reveals an echogenic density
causing acoustic shadowing just at the neck of the gallbladder (Fig. 2-27, arrow).
This appearance was reproducible on many longitudinal scans.

FOLLOW UP

At surgery, gallstones and cystic duct stones were found.

COMMENT

The problem of cystic duct stones has received scant attention in the literature. Anderson and Harned have referred to this diagnosis in a recent review of
gallbladder sonography.[1] Experience has shown, however, that shadowing at the
neck of the gallbladder is occasionally seen in normal patients (Fig. 2-28).

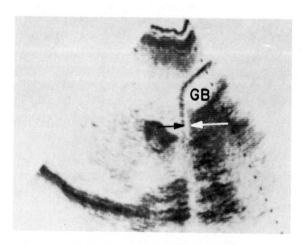

**Fig. 2-28.**   Longitudinal scan.  Note shadow (arrows) at
neck of gallbladder.

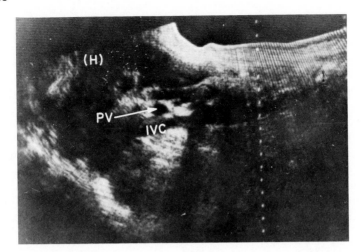

**Fig. 2-29.** Longitudinal scan. A branch of the portal vein (PV) and IVC are labeled.

On occasion, however, a discrete echogenic density at the gallbladder neck may be traced to the acoustic shadow and may strongly suggest a cystic duct stone. Associated findings, such as gallstones and a tender, dilated gallbladder, help to elevate one's confidence in making this diagnosis.

### Case

TS is a 52-year-old female with mild right upper quadrant pain and jaundice. She had a cholecystectomy five years prior to admission. Representative longitudinal and transverse sections of the upper abdomen are shown in Fig. 2-29, 2-30. Since the gallbladder has been removed in the past, we are, of course, looking at other portions of the biliary tree, such as the common bile duct. Is the common duct dilated, and, if so, can you identify the cause of the obstruction?

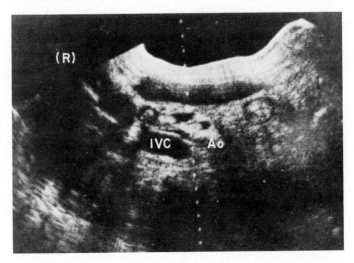

**Fig. 2-30.** Transverse scan of epigastrium. The aorta (Ao) and IVC are labeled.

## DISCUSSION

Referring to the longitudinal semidecubitus scan in Fig. 2-31, a tubular structure passing just over the portal vein (large arrows) can be identified. This is a dilated common bile duct measuring approximately 12 mm in diameter. Since the common duct runs in an oblique direction as it passes caudally, only portions of the duct are seen on the longitudinal scans. With a real time system, it is a simple matter to follow this structure by turning the transducer until the bulk of the common duct is seen. With a sector scanner, a more difficult maneuver is needed, as the patient has to be oblique to accomplish the same goal. The importance of visualizing as much of the common bile duct as possible becomes apparent as Fig.2-31 is examined more critically. Within the duct there is an echogenic density (small arrows) associated with an acoustic shadow. This stone can also be identified within the cross-sectional lumen of the common duct (Fig. 2-32, arrow).

## FOLLOW UP

A transhepatic cholangiogram was performed (Fig. 2-33) and revealed a dilated common bile duct with an obstructing stone (arrow).

## COMMENTS

1.  The common bile duct may be a difficult structure to visualize sonographically. Experience has shown that the best way to identify this structure is by performing longitudinal semidecubitus scans with the patient slightly oblique so that the transducer passes from right to left as it sweeps caudally. Careful scanning may reveal not only a dilated common duct but stones within the

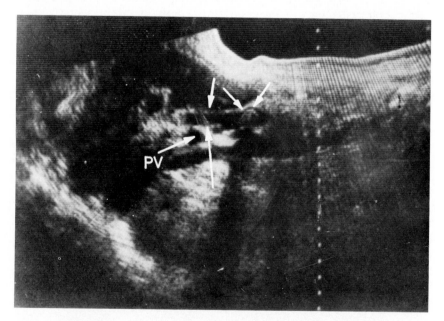

**Fig. 2-31.** Longitudinal scan. Note dilated common bile duct (large arrows) passing over a branch of the portal vein (PV). There is an echogenic density within the CBD (small arrows) associated with an acoustic shadow.

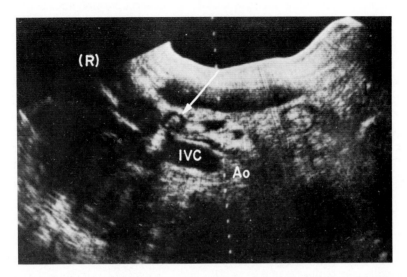

**Fig. 2-32.** Transverse scan. Note echogenic density (arrow) within the dilated common bile duct.

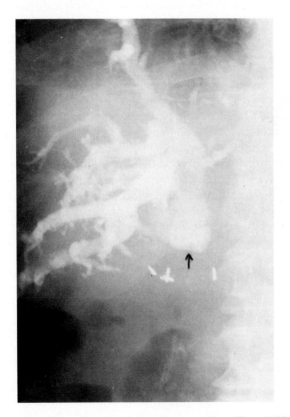

**Fig. 2-33.** Transhepatic cholangiogram. Note dilated biliary tree secondary to an obstructing stone (arrow).

duct. The failure to find stones within the dilated common duct certainly does not rule out this possibility. Because of the course of this structure, the entire duct may not be visualized. Moreover, stones near the ampulla may be obscured by gas within the duodenum.

2.  Sonography of the common bile duct may serve as an effective alternative to conventional studies such as oral cholecystography and intravenous cholangiography in two categories of patients: (1) those with elevated serum bilirubin levels in whom conventional studies are not possible and (2) those who have had previous cholecystectomies. Oral cholecystography, of course, cannot be performed in these patients, who may be screened with a sonographic examination. If the common bile duct and stones are visualized as in this case, further evaluation may not be necessary.


## SUMMARY

A complete gallbladder sonogram should include visualization of other organs, such as the pancreas and liver. Of course, views of the gallbladder in several different planes and positions are also required. We have found the longitudinal semidecubitus scan to be the most effective in the identification of gallstones.

The classic gallstone fulfills three criteria. It is (1) a discrete echogenic density, (2) within a fluid-filled gallbladder, and (3) causes acoustic shadowing. A vast majority of stones fulfill all three criteria. Aside from gas, shadowing in the right upper quadrant may be due to a gallbladder filled with stones, or a porcelain gallbladder. The latter two entities present sonographically as discrete echogenic densities associated with sharply defined acoustic shadows. A normal fluid-filled gallbladder cannot be found. The conventional x-ray examination, KUB, distinguishes the "packed bag" from the porcelain gallbladder.

Cystic duct stones appear sonographically as discrete echogenic, shadowcasting densities at the neck of the gallbladder. Care must be taken because shadowing is occasionally identified at the neck of normal gallbladders.

With careful scanning, the common bile duct and stones within the duct may be identified. Again, the longitudinal semidecubitus scan has been found to be the most effective. Sonographic cholecystography may be a useful alternative to intravenous cholangiography, especially in jaundiced patients. It should be remembered, however, that failure to find sonographic evidence of a stone does not rule out the existence of such a stone.


## REFERENCES

1.  Anderson JC, Harned RK: Gray scale ultrasonography of the gallbladder: An evaluation of accuracy and report of additional ultrasound signs. Am J Roentgenol 129:975–977, 1977
2.  Arnon S, Rosenquist CJ: Gray scale cholecystosonography: An evaluation of accuracy. Am J Roentgenol 127:817–818, 1976
3.  Bartrum RJ: Ultrasound examination of the gallbladder. JAMA 235:1147–1148, 1976
4.  Goldberg BB: Ultrasonic cholangiography. Radiology 118:401–403, 1976

5.  Hublitz UF, Kahn PC, Sall LA: Cholecystosonography; an approach to the nonvisualized gallbladder. Radiology 103:645–649, 1972

6.  Leopold GR, Amberg J, Gosink BB, et al: Gray scale cholecystography: A comparison with conventional radiographic techniques. Radiology 121:445–448, 1976

7.  Thal ER, Weigelt J, Landay M, et al: Evaluation of ultrasound in the diagnosis of acute and chronic biliary tract disease. Arch Surg 113:500–503, 1978

8.  Kappelman NB, Sanders RC: Ultrasound in the investigation of gallbladder disease. JAMA 239:1426–1428, 1978

9.  Goldberg BB (ed): Abdominal gray scale ultrasonography. New York, Wiley, 1977, p 149

10. Ibid, p 59

11. Taylor KJW, Carpenter BE, McCready VR: Ultrasound and scintigraphy in the differential diagnosis of obstructive jaundice. J Clin Ultrasound 2:105–116, 1974

12. Conrad MR, Landay MJ, Jones JO: Sonographic "parallel channel" sign of biliary tree enlargement in mild to moderate obstructive jaundice. Am J Roentgenol 130: 279–286, 1978

# 3

# The Dilated Gallbladder

As a result of the new window into the right upper quadrant that ultrasound provides, abnormalities never before appreciated now need explanation. One such abnormality is the dilated gallbladder. The logical question that one might ask at this point is, "Just how large does a gallbladder have to be to be considered dilated?" Goldberg describes a dilated gallbladder as being greater than 8 cm in length and 3.5 to 4 cm in width.[1] But measurements have not correlated very well. What measures out to be an enlarged gallbladder in a small patient may be perfectly normal in a large patient. My only answer is that I think I know an enlarged gallbladder when I see one. Since this is not a very illuminating description, several illustrative cases have been reproduced. On sagittal sections, the dilated gallbladder assumes a very impressive elongated appearance within the right upper quadrant (Figs. 3-1A, 3-1B).

On transverse sections, the cross-sectional lumen of the gallbladder fills a large percentage of the right anterior quadrant (Fig. 3-2)

The dilated gallbladder may become apparent to the sonographer in several situations besides gallbladder sonography. While one is evaluating other organs, such as the liver, pancreas, kidneys, and aorta, the dilated gallbladder may be shouting for recognition. Once it is discovered, it must be explained. It may, indeed, be normal. It may also be a signal of occult pathology, such as carcinoma of the pancreas.

We have found it useful to classify the etiology of gallbladder distention into the following categories:


   I   Normal variant—contracts after a fatty meal
  II  Associated with an obstructing stone
      A. Cystic duct
      B. Common bile duct
 III  Associated with an obstructing mass
 IV  Associated with no visualized obstructing stone or mass

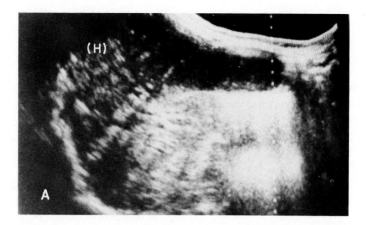

**Fig. 3-1 A.** Supine, longitudinal scan. Note dilated GB with debris.

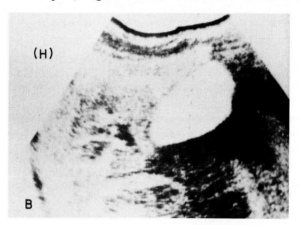

**Fig. 3-1 B.** Supine, longitudinal scan showing dilated GB.

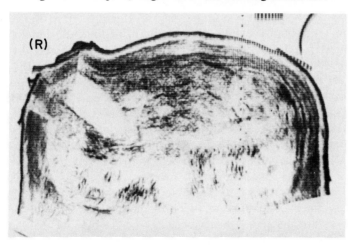

**Fig. 3-2.** Supine, transverse scan.

After an apparently dilated gallbladder is discovered, the case should be fitted into one of the first three categories. If this is unsuccessful, the case must be placed into the waste paper basket category IV. Each of these categories will be discussed in detail as illustrative cases are presented.

There are a few general principles regarding dilated gallbladders. First, in cases where there is partial obstruction of the common bile duct, the gallbladder may become dilated before other components of the biliary tree. Indeed, gallbladder dilatation may even precede the onset of appreciable increase in the serum bilirubin level. Because of its unique physical properties, the gallbladder is usually the first component of the biliary tree to respond to early increases in pressure secondary to obstruction by stricture, stone, or mass. To explain this phenomenon, it may be useful to refer to a paper published by Compton in 1973, in which Compton attempted to apply physical principles to hollow organs within the body —ureters, renal pelvis, cecum, and so on. He states, "The following may thus apply to all hollow organs: For a given uniform positive pressure throughout a fluid-filled organ or viscus, the force tending to cause a dilation or bursting is the greatest at the site of the greatest radius."[2] Within the biliary tree, including the gallbladder, small biliary ducts, common duct, and cystic duct, the gallbladder is certainly the site of greatest radius and is usually the organ that responds first to early pressure changes within the biliary tree, provided, of course, that there is no preexisting inflammatory fibrosis of the gallbladder. The gallbladder, therefore, may serve as the earliest indicator of obstruction of the common bile duct.

The second general principle is based on the often quoted Courvoisier Law. In essence, the nineteenth century surgeon stated that, in patients with jaundice, the physical finding of a palpable, dilated gallbladder suggests the diagnosis of carcinoma of the pancreas.[3] The rationale behind this statement is based primarily on the fact that the other major cause of a dilated gallbladder, an obstructing stone, would be associated with preexisting inflammatory disease of the gallbladder. The walls of the gallbladder would, therefore, be fibrosed and incapable of dilatation. Now that we are in a better position to appreciate the dilated gallbladder by means of ultrasound, we have found that, as a law, Courvoisier's observation does not hold true in many circumstances.

If the law is analyzed, two assumptions are apparent. First, that carcinoma of the pancreatic head is associated with dilatation of the gallbladder. In the vast majority of cases, this assumption has been found to be true. Indeed, as mentioned above, the gallbladder is frequently the first component of the biliary tree to dilate when the common bile duct is obstructed. It is the second assumption that is debatable—that preexisting inflammatory disease of the gallbladder renders it incapable of distention. Experience has shown that this has not been the case. Many cases of dilated gallbladders with stones associated with a number of etiologies have been seen, including cystic and common bile duct stones, carcinoma of the common bile duct, metastatic disease in the *porta hepatis*, as well as carcinoma of the pancreas. Preexisting inflammatory disease as manifested by the presence of gallstones does not appear to render the gallbladder indistensible, although there are occasional cases in which the walls of the gallbladder cannot respond to pressure changes within the biliary tree. Even in view of the seemingly endless violations of the law, it serves a very useful purpose—it alerts the sonographer/physician to the possibility of carcinoma of the pancreas as the underlying cause of the dilated gallbladder.

### Case

HR is a 35-year-old, asymptomatic male, who has fasted for approximately 16 hours. A longitudinal prelunch scan is reproduced below in Fig. 3-3. Approximately 45 to 60 minutes after lunch in the hospital cafeteria, the scan reveals significant contraction of the gallbladder (Fig. 3-4).

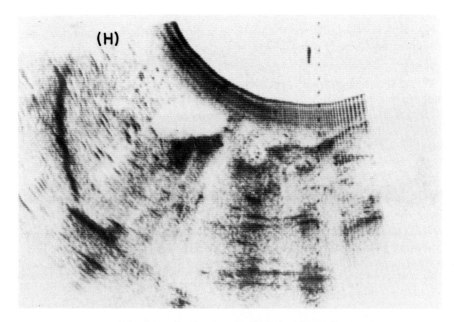

**Fig. 3-3.** Supine longitudinal "prelunch" scan.

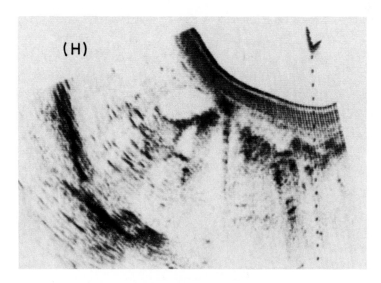

**Fig. 3-4.** Supine longitudinal "postlunch" scan.

DISCUSSION

The patient, of course, is myself, and to avoid the biliary colic that results from such forceful contraction of my gallbladder, I limit my attendance at the hospital cafeteria. The scan, however, does demonstrate the value of a fatty meal in normal patients with enlarged fasting gallbladders. It should be mentioned that the fatty meal is only a rough approximation of the gallbladder's ability to contract. Prior to the fatty meal, attempts are made to obtain the maximum longitudinal and transverse diameters and these scans are repeated about one hour after the meal.

FOLLOW UP

No surgical proof. The patient is alive and well and able to eat a hot pastrami sandwich without severe aftereffects.

COMMENTS

This case is a somewhat facetious example of category I. The success or lack of success that one may have with fatty meals depends on the type of stimulant used, technique, and other factors. Some authors have success, others do not. I personally feel that the the test is useful if, and only if, very rigid controls are used.

### Case

RN is a 57-year-old- male who had had a partial colonic resection for carcinoma of the sigmoid four years before this admission. A radionuclide liver scan (Fig. 3-5) revealed a defect along the inferior surface of the right lobe, probably representing gallbladder bed. Pre- and post-fatty meal, longitudinal scans and a transverse scan are shown below and opposite (Fig. 3-6, 3-7, 3-8). Do you think that the gallbladder accounts for the defect on the liver scan? Are there any clues as to why the gallbladder is enlarged?

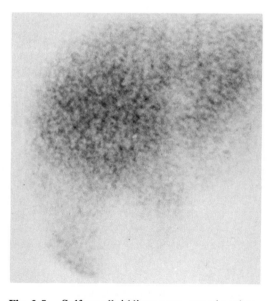

**Fig. 3-5.**  Sulfur colloid liver scan, anterior view.

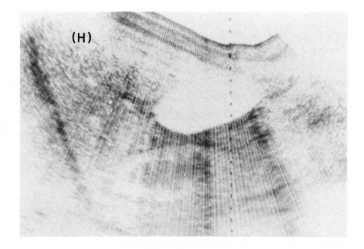

**Fig. 3-6.** Longitudinal pre-fatty meal scan.

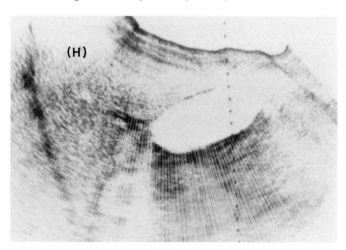

**Fig 3-7.** Longitudinal post-fatty meal scan.

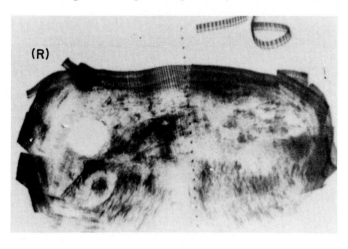

**Fig. 3-8.** Transverse scan.

DISCUSSION

   The pre-fatty meal scan reveals a dilated gallbladder (Fig. 3-9). There is an acoustic shadow (arrows) associated with a density at the neck of the gallbladder which probably represents a cystic duct stone. A post-fatty meal scan reveals no significant contraction of the gallbladder. One knows, therefore, that one is not dealing with an enlarged gallbladder as a normal variant. The transverse scan (Fig. 3-10) reveals a dilated gallbladder, most probably accounting for the defect on the liver scan. These scans and others not reproduced revealed no evidence of enlarged common bile duct, biliary radicles, or a pancreatic mass.

FOLLOW UP

   An intravenous cholangiogram revealed a common bile duct of normal caliber. There was no visualization of the gallbladder or cystic duct. At surgery, an enlarged gallbladder with a stone impacted in the cystic duct was found (Fig. 3-11).

COMMENTS

1.   In the past, attempts at evaluation of the gallbladder defect on the liver scan consisted of rose bengal scans and oral cholecystography. Ultrasound now provides a more rapid and effective means of providing this information.
2.   Referring to the classification of dilated gallbladders on page 49, it can be seen that this case falls into category IIA. The cystic duct stone that is identified on

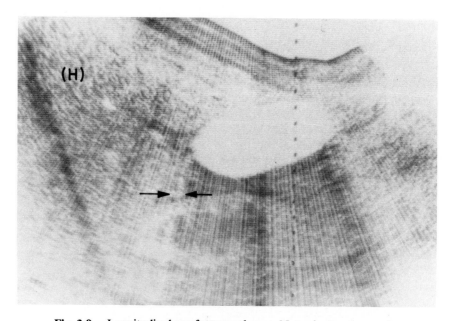

**Fig. 3-9.**   Longitudinal pre-fatty meal scan. Note shadow (arrows).

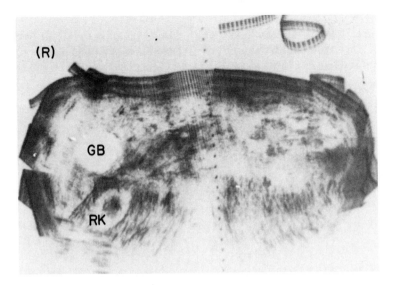

**Fig 3-10.**  Transverse scan showing dilated gallbladder.

the sonograms is fairly convincing, but not quite convincing enough to make a definitive diagnosis. As mentioned in the preceeding chapter, shadowing is occasionally seen at the neck of normal gallbladders. Reassured by the findings of the intravenous cholangiogram, in further questioning of the patient we did learn that he had had a recent onset of right upper quadrant pain. The history tended to place the pathology in a category where one would expect acute symptoms such as occur with cystic duct stones.

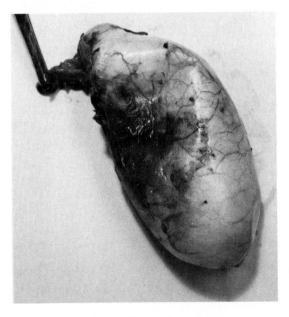

**Fig. 3-11.**  Surgical specimen.

**Case**

LB is a 35-year-old female admitted with right upper quadrant pain and mild jaundice, whose gallbladder sonogram is reproduced below (Fig.3-12, 3-13, 3-14). What is your diagnosis? In which of the four categories would you put this case?

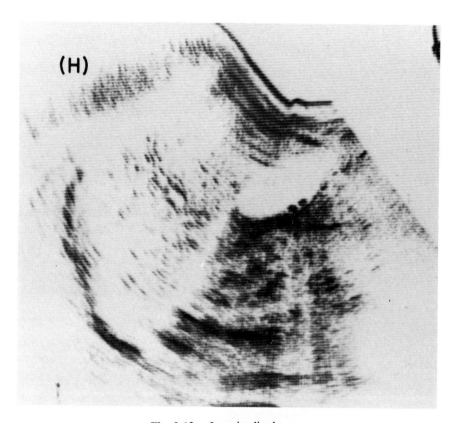

**Fig. 3-12.**   Longitudinal scan.

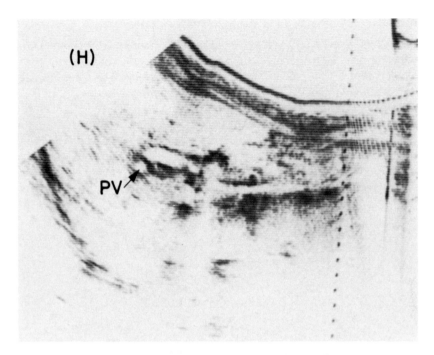

**Fig. 3-13.**   Longitudinal scan. The portal vein (PV) is labeled.

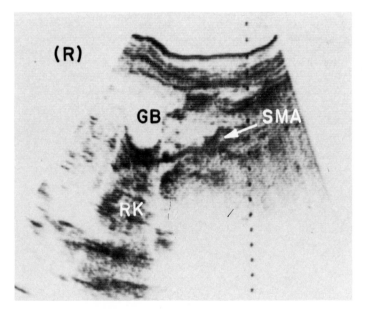

**Fig. 3-14.**   Transverse scan. The right kidney (RK), gallbladder (GB), and superior mesenteric artery (SMA) are labeled.

DISCUSSION

Again, this is a dilated gallbladder (Fig.3-12). Stones are present within the gallbladder lumen. Because of the patient's clinical and sonographic picture, it was decided that a fatty meal would not be necessary. The longitudinal semi-decubitus scan (Fig. 3-15A) reveals a dilated common bile duct (CBD) passing over the cross-sectional lumen of the portal vein (PV). There is a discrete echogenic density within the common duct (arrow). There is no associated shadow, but the stone is small and at a level in the scan where a shadow would be difficult to appreciate. Compare this scan to a section taken 1 cm more to the right (Fig. 3-15B). The common bile duct is dilated, but there is no evidence of a stone.

The dilated common bile duct and stone can also be identified on the trans-

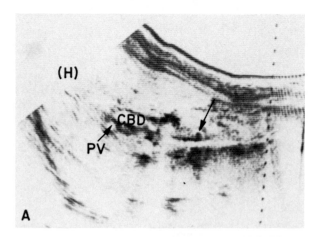

**Fig. 3-15 A.** Longitudinal scan. The dilated common bile duct (CBD) passes over the portal vein (PV). A small echogenic density is noted within the common bile duct (arrow).

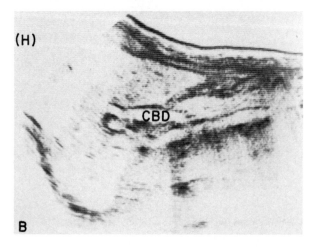

**Fig. 3-15 B.** Longitudinal scan. The dilated CBD is well seen. The stone is not present on this section.

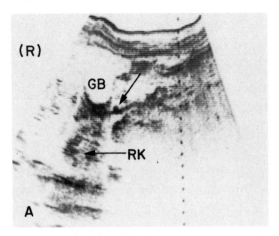

**Fig. 3-16 A.**    Transverse scan. Note stone within CBD (arrow).

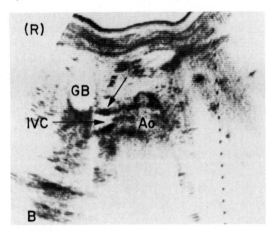

**Fig. 3-16 B.**    Transverse scan. This scan was taken at 0.5 cm. cephalad to Fig. 3-16 A. A dilated CBD (arrow) is noted, but the stone is not present.

verse sections (Fig. 3-16A, arrow). Another scan (Fig. 3-16B) 0.5 cm cephalad to the scan in Fig. 16A, reveals a dilated common bile duct (arrow). The stone cannot be seen at this level.

FOLLOW UP

At surgery, a dilated common bile duct with multiple stones was found.

COMMENTS

Finding the dilated common bile duct is generally not a serious problem. Conrad and associates have described a sign of biliary tree enlargement in cases of mild-to-moderate obstructive jaundice.[4] The so-called parallel channel sign is a result of simultaneous imaging of the hepatic ducts with adjacent branches of the

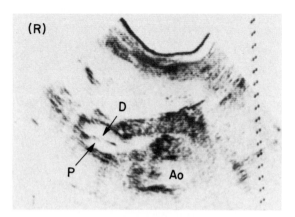

**Fig. 3-17.** Transverse scan of epigastrium. The contiguous common bile duct (CBD) and branch of the portal vein (P) resulting in the "parallel channel."

portal vein. Above is an example (Fig. 3-17). The common bile duct (CBD) lies just anterior to a branch of the portal vein (P).

Finding a stone in the common duct requires very diligent scanning. At best, the findings are subtle. In this case, as in the preceding case, we were reassured by the patient's age and acute nature of her symptoms. When there is doubt, further evaluation, such as transhepatic cholangiography, should be considered.

### Case

AB is a 74-year-old male with jaundice and mild right upper quadrant pain. Representative longitudinal scans are reproduced below and opposite (Figs. 3-18, 3-19, 3-20, 3-21). What portions of the biliary tree are dilated? Can you identify the cause of obstruction?

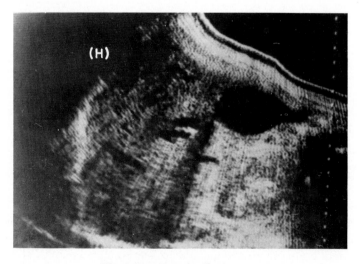

**Fig. 3-18.** Longitudinal scan.

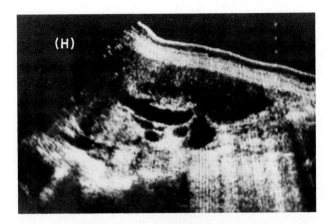

**Fig. 3-19.** Longitudinal scan.

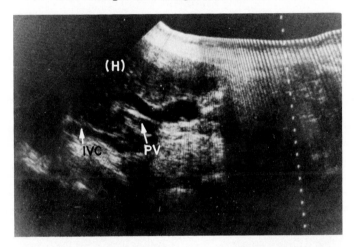

**Fig. 3-20.** Longitudinal scan. The IVC and portal vein (PV) are labeled.

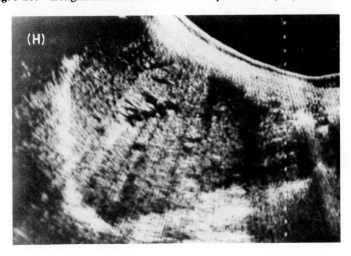

**Fig. 3-21.** Longitudinal scan.

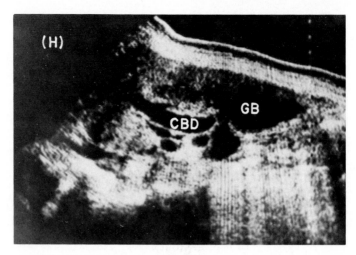

**Fig. 3-22.**    Longitudinal scan revealing dilated gallbladder and CBD.

DISCUSSION

The longitudinal scan reveals a dilated gallbladder, common bile duct (Fig. 3-22), and biliary radicles (Fig. 3-23, arrows). In addition to identifying the dilated biliary tree, it was thought that a stone in the common bile duct could be seen (Fig. 3-24, arrow). Admittedly, this is not a definitive finding. Because of gas, the common duct on the transverse sections was not identified, and no evidence of a pancreatic or *porta* mass was seen.

FOLLOW UP

Since there was uncertainty of the stone, a transhepatic cholangiogram (Fig. 3-25) was performed. The common bile duct was dilated and at the site of obstruc-

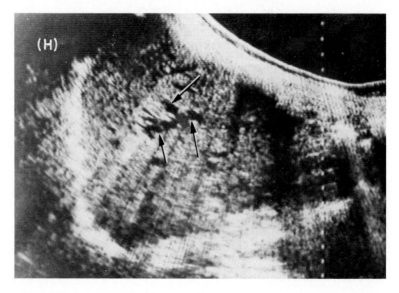

**Fig. 3-23.**    Longitudinal scan revealing dilated biliary ducts (arrows).

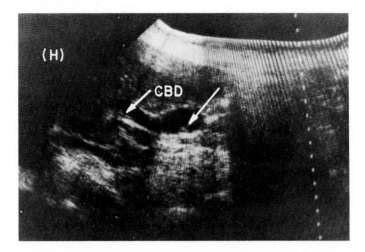

**Fig. 3-24.** Longitudinal scan revealing dilated CBD and stone (arrow).

tion there was a concave defect suggesting an impacted stone (arrow). These findings were confirmed at surgery.

COMMENTS

This case serves as an introduction to category IV. Category III will be considered in more detail in the next chapter. Category IV has two distinctions. First, when a case falls into this group, the etiology of the gallbladder distention is uncertain and, in general, requires further evaluation. Second, it is unfortunate that, with existing equipment, many cases fall into this category. No doubt as technology improves with digital scan converters and real time instrumentation, greater accuracy will be attained in the assessment of biliary stones and right

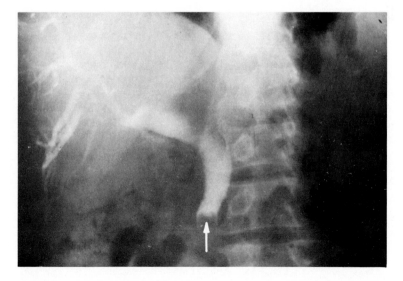

**Fig. 3-25.** Transhepatic cholangiogram. Note obstructing stone (arrow).

upper quadrant masses. At present, cases fall into the uncertain category IV and require additional evaluation.

Studies such as upper GI series and intravenous cholangiography remain very important modalities in the evaluation of obstructive jaundice. Direct visualization of the biliary tree can be accomplished by means of transhepatic cholangiography. This examination has received widespread acceptance. The study is relatively easy to perform with a skinny needle. The examination, when performed correctly, yields very useful information concerning the presence of stones in the common bile duct, primary tumors of the common duct, and adjacent tumors, such as carcinoma of the pancreatic head. With certain exceptions that will be pointed out later, transhepatic cholangiograms are routinely performed in cases that fall into category IV.

### Case

JS is a 52-year-old male who presented with weight loss, jaundice, and epigastric pain. A radionuclide liver scan is shown below (Fig. 3-26). Opposite are representative sagittal scans of the right upper quadrant (Fig. 3-27, 3-28, 3-29). Given these studies, what would you conclude and what further workup would you recommend?

**Fig. 3-26.**   Sulfur colloid liver scan.

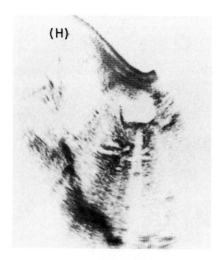

**Fig. 3-27.** Longitudinal scan.

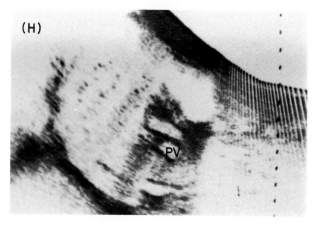

**Fig. 3-28.** Longitudinal scan. The portal vein (PV) is labeled.

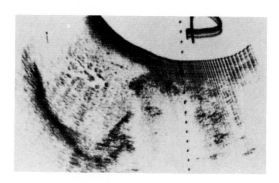

**Fig. 3-29.** Longitudinal scan.

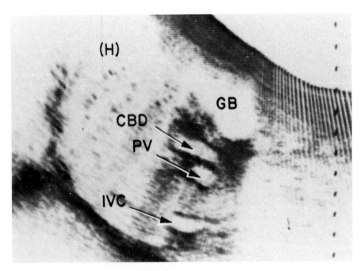

**Fig. 3-30.** Longitudinal scan. Note dilated CBD, GB. The portal vein (PV), and a small portion of the IVC are labeled.

## DISCUSSION

The liver scan is suggestive of a dilated biliary tree, a finding that is confirmed by sonography. The gallbladder, common bile duct (Fig. 3-30), and the biliary radicles (Fig. 3-31, arrows) are dilated. Gallstones are present (Fig. 3-27). There was no evidence of a pancreatic mass.

## FOLLOW UP

It was elected to do a transhepatic cholangiogram (Fig. 3-32). An area of irregular narrowing was identified, involving the midportion of the common duct (arrows). A similar pattern in the large bowel would be pathognomonic of carcinoma. The preoperative diagnosis of carcinoma of the common bile duct was made, which was confirmed at surgery.

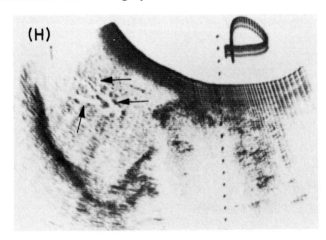

**Fig. 3-31.** Longitudinal scan revealing dilated biliary ducts (arrows).

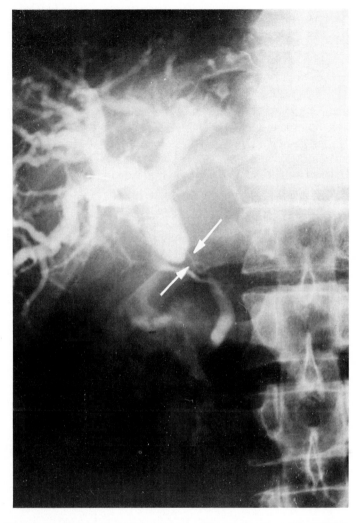

**Fig. 3-32.** Transhepatic cholangiogram revealing narrowing of the CBD (arrows).

COMMENTS

1. This case falls into the uncertain category IV, and points out the importance of transhepatic cholangiography in making a definitive diagnosis. With existing ultrasound equipment, it would be difficult to demonstrate carcinoma of the common duct. When dealing with tubular organs, common sense dictates that the best way of visualizing such structures would be to put in contrast material. The sonogram did, however, tell us that we were dealing with extrahepatic obstruction. It remained for the transhepatic cholangiogram to indicate the nature of the obstruction. Frequently, as was seen and will be seen in later cases in the book, the level of obstruction (categories IIB, III) can be identified.

2. JS did have gallstones as demonstrated in Fig. 3-27. Should the presence of

gallstones have made one suspicious of an impacted bile duct stone? One thinks not. The presence of gallstones means very little, being very common and possibly associated with anything, including carcinoma of the pancreas, carcinoma of the common duct, or a bunion, for that matter. Gallstones should be treated as incidental, rather than causative, findings in cases such as this.

There are, however, certain clues that can help one out of the muddle of category IV. In essence, one is dealing with either acute inflammatory disease and stones, or occult neoplasm. The symptoms that JS had were of a relatively long duration and were associated with weight loss. We were not, therefore, surprised at the results of the transhepatic cholangiogram.

### Case

JR is a 52-year-old male who presented with severe right upper quadrant pain. A KUB(Fig. 3-33, below) revealed a large soft tissue mass in the right side of the abdomen, extending down below the iliac crest. Supine, longitudinal, and transverse scans are shown opposite (Fig. 3-34, 3-35, 3-36). On the basis of these scans, how would you explain the mass seen on the KUB?

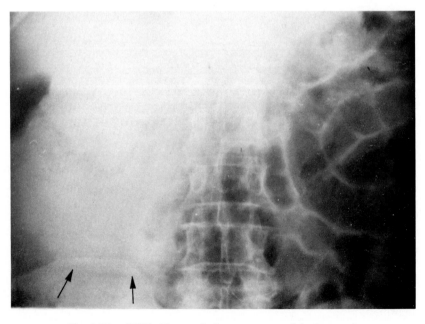

**Fig. 3-33.**   KUB. Note soft tissue mass on right (arrows).

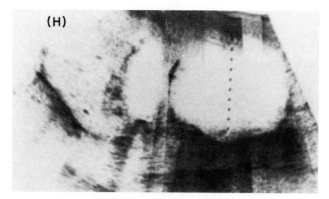

**Fig. 3-34.** Longitudinal scan.

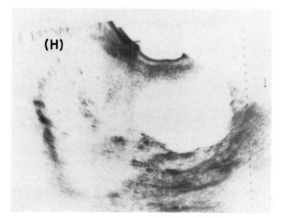

**Fig. 3-35.** Longitudinal scan 2 cm. to the right of the scan in Fig. 3-34.

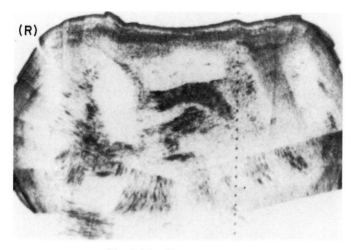

**Fig. 3-36.** Transverse scan.

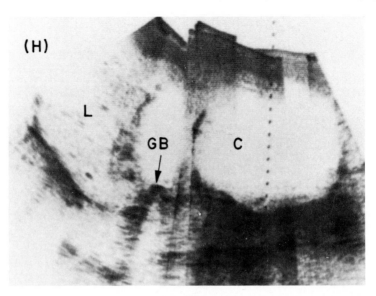

**Fig. 3-37.** Longitudinal scan. The liver (L), GB, stone (arrow), and cyst (C) are labeled.

DISCUSSION

The scan reproduced in Fig. 3-37 is a confusing picture. It is usually helpful to begin with portions of the anatomy that are known. The scan is a longitudinal section of the right upper quadrant, with the right hemidiaphragm and liver parenchyma serving as useful landmarks. Just below the liver (L) there is an elliptical sonolucent mass which represents an enlarged gallbladder (GB). An echogenic shadow-casting density is noted within the neck of the gallbladder which represents a stone (arrow). Another larger sonolucent mass is identified adjacent to the gallbladder. The longitudinal scan just lateral to the gallbladder (Fig. 3-38), shows that the mass (C) arises from the anterior aspect of the right kidney (RK) and probably represents a renal cyst.

The transverse scan (Fig. 3-39) reveals a dilated gallbladder (GB), gallstone (arrow), and right renal cyst (C). Other scans, not shown, revealed no evidence of pancreatic mass or dilated biliary tree. It was concluded that the patient had an empyema of the gallbladder, probably secondary to cystic duct obstruction. This conclusion was based principally on the following observations: (1) enlarged, palpable, tender gallbladder, (2) no evidence of dilatation of other portions of the biliary tree, (3) no evidence of a pancreatic mass.

FOLLOW UP

At surgery, an empyema of the gallbladder secondary to cystic duct obstruction was found. A large right renal cyst was also encountered.

COMMENTS

1.  This case demonstrates the importance of palpation during the sonographic examination. Our staff members hold the ultrasound transducer near the con-

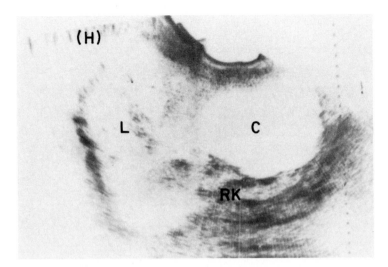

**Fig. 3-38.**   Longitudinal scan revealing cyst (C) arising from right kidney (RK).

tact surface and, as a result, they are in an excellent position to palpate the abdomen while watching the television screen. They are simultaneously aware of the palpatory and sonographic findings. In this case, for example, a tense mass was freely palpable in the right upper quadrant, and one knew that the mass represented the gallbladder by simply watching the screen (Fig. 3-40). In the same manner, it could be seen that the patient had exquisite tenderness when the gallbladder was palpated.

2.  Since certain identification of the cause of gallbladder distention was not possible, this case falls into category IV. The stone that was identified lies at the neck of the gallbladder near the cystic duct. The right renal cyst distorts

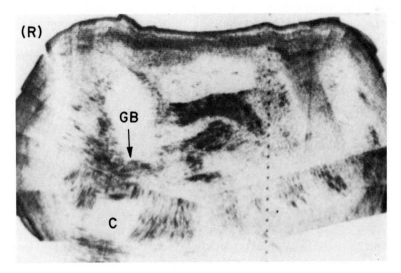

**Fig. 3-39.**   Transverse scan. Note dilated gallbladder with stone (arrow) and right renal cyst (C).

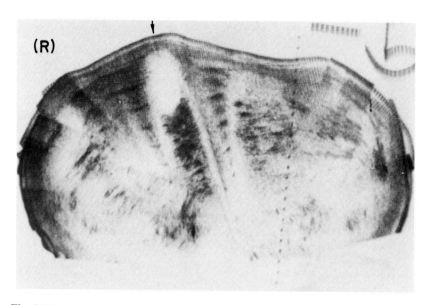

**Fig. 3-40.** Transverse scan. The dilated gallbladder was easily palpable (arrow).

the anatomy enough to confuse the picture. As had been suspected prior to surgery, the cyst was adjacent to the gallbladder and pushed it up against the liver. The gallbladder neck, consequently, was difficult to evaluate.

This is another case in which the clinical picture helped us out of the uncertainty of category IV. Technically, as mentioned previously, a transhepatic cholangiogram should have followed. But this case, and others like it, are exceptions. The severity of the patient's symptoms superseded further investigations. This patient was acutely ill, febrile, and had marked pinpoint tenderness over the gallbladder. The acute nature of the symptoms made it likely that inflammatory disease was present, and the absence of common duct enlargement tended to localize the level of pathology to the gallbladder and cystic duct. Although we did not reach the high level of confidence that a transhepatic cholangiogram would have afforded, we were reasonably confident in our diagnosis.

## SUMMARY

The following is a summary of the categories of dilated gallbladders considered in this chapter.

*Category I.* Normal variant. A rigidly controlled fatty meal challenge helps in isolating this gallbladder from the pathologic states discussed below.

*Category IIA.* Cystic duct obstruction secondary to a stone. As mentioned in Chapter 2, cystic duct stones appear sonographically as discrete echogenic, shadow-casting densities at the neck of the gallbladder. Care must be taken because shadowing is occasionally identified at the neck of normal gallbladders.

*Category IIB.* Common bile duct stones. With careful scanning, the common bile duct and stones within may be identified. Intravenous or transhepatic cholangiography are useful studies when there is doubt concerning the presence of common duct stones.

*Category III.* Sonographic evidence of an obstructing pancreatic or *porta* mass. This category will be discussed in the next chapter.

*Category IV.* No sonographic evidence of an obstructing stone or mass. This is the waste paper basket category, and cases that fall into it need further evaluation. Transhepatic cholangiography has been found to be very helpful. A clinical picture that is acute suggests inflammatory disease with stones, while a long-standing history suggests neoplasm involving the common duct or adjacent structures.

The gallbladder may be the first indicator of increasing pressure within the biliary system by dilating before other components, such as the common bile duct and biliary radicles. Indeed, the dilated gallbladder may become apparent before any increase in the serum bilirubin level is appreciated. For this reason, it is essential to investigate these cases and eliminate the possibilities of obstructing masses or stones.

**REFERENCES**

1.  Goldberg BB: Abdominal Gray Scale Ultrasonography. New York, Wiley, 1977, p 144–145
2.  Compton RA: Bursting forces within the human body. Radiology 107:77–80, 1973
3.  Bailey H: Notable Names in Medicine and Surgery. London, HK Lewis, 1949, pp 135–137
4.  Conrad MR, Landay MJ, Jones JO, Sonographic ''parallel channel'' sign of biliary tree enlargement in mild to moderate obstructive jaundice. Am J Roentgenol. 130:274–286, 1978

# 4

# Pancreas

The pancreas, up to very recently, has been one of the most difficult organs to evaluate by imaging systems. Principal reliance has been on studying the effects that this gland has on the barium-filled upper gastrointestinal tract, especially the duodenum. Arteriography has been useful, but not as a screening procedure. Radionuclide imaging has proved to be disappointing. Ultrasound, endoscopic retrograde catheterization of the pancreatic duct (ERCP), and computerized scanning have provided much more realistic and accurate modalities to evaluate this occult organ.

Recent and current on-going studies are examining the relative merits of each of these examinations. At present, pancreatic sonography has received the most widespread acceptance. Equipment required is less costly than that required for computerized body scanning and, as compared to ERCP, is totally noninvasive.

For several reasons, pancreatic sonography remains one of the most difficult ultrasound examinations to perform and interpret. First, gas frequently obscures areas of the abdomen that are critical for evaluation of the pancreas. This is especially true of the body and tail, but of the head as well. Premedication with simethicone has not proved to be successful at our institution. An adequate study on certain patients simply cannot be performed, no matter what preparations are used, or how many times the study is attempted. Patients with conditions such as acute pancreatitis frequently have reflex distention of portions of their small and large bowels. Thus, an unfortunate paradox is established—the patients whom one is most eager to study are the ones that are most difficult because of the presence of gas. Occasionally, the semidecubitus position described in Chapter 2 may be helpful.

Second, even when a perfect sonic window is available, the pancreas is a difficult organ to visualize. Its distribution is very tortuous and variable. Moreover, its ultrasonic characteristics, although not identical, are similar to surrounding structures such as the liver. Because of these difficulties, the sonographer must be intimately aware of the anatomic relations of adjacent structures such as the inferior vena cava, aorta, and so forth.

## INDICATIONS

In many institutions, pancreatic sonography frequently serves as a front-line investigative procedure in the following situations:

1. Clinical picture and/or laboratory findings suggestive of acute pancreatitis.
2. Patients with pancreatitis in whom follow-up studies are required for evaluation of the pancreas and question of pseudocyst formation.
3. Follow-up evaluation of a pseudocyst.
4. Patients in whom carcinoma of the pancreas may be suspected.

As a secondary study, pancreatic sonography is used to:

1. Rule out the presence of edema or mass in the pancreatic head after suspicion is raised by an abnormal duodenum on upper GI series.
2. Rule out the presence of a pancreatic mass causing obstruction of the common bile duct and a dilated gallbladder.

## TECHNIQUE

The abdominal sonogram described in Chapter 1 serves as the backbone of the pancreatic study. Attention is then focused on the epigastrium, and very detailed scans of this area are obtained. The transverse scans are single pass, limited sector sweeps, performed in maximal inspiration. No attempt is made to complete the scan by compounding around the lateral aspects of the abdomen. The completed scans are included in the basic abdominal study and provide useful gross anatomic information. The information required in the epigastrium, however, is very detailed, and compounding may obliterate some of the detail obtained in the limited sector scan.

The problem of gas obscuring important epigastric structures may occasionally be solved by using the following technique. The transducer arm is angled approximately 10 degrees toward the patient's feet. The sound beam passes in a slightly caudal angle. As a result, the left lobe of the liver serves as an acoustic window through which the important structures in the epigastrium may be visualized.

Using this technique, a plethora of structures may be identified. The area of interest is bordered by the liver on the right and by gas in the stomach on the left. Below, the basic vascular anatomy relative to the pancreas is outlined. It is not within the scope of this book to present a detailed description of these structures in the upper abdomen. For this information, the reader is referred to the bibliography at the end of Chapter 1, as well as to the excellent chapter on this subject written by Filly and Goldberg in *Abdominal Gray Scale Ultrasonography*.[1]

## SONOANATOMY

The following structures may be identified on the transverse scans:

*Splenic vein.* The venous phases of celiac (Fig.4-1) and superior mesenteric (Fig.4-2) arteriograms demonstrate the course of the splenic (S), superior mesen-

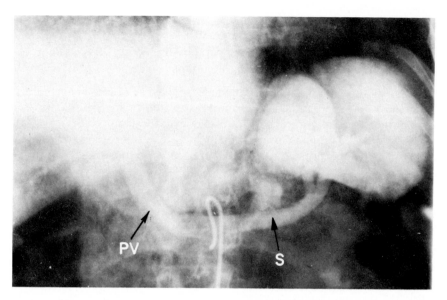

**Fig. 4-1.** Venous phase of celiac arteriogram. Note splenic (S) and portal (PV) veins.

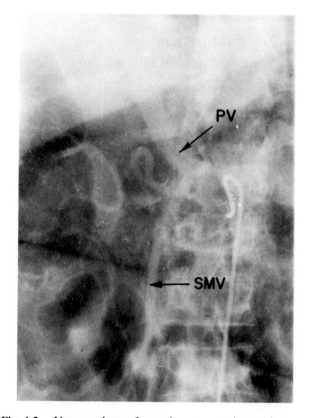

**Fig. 4-2.** Venous phase of superior mesenteric arteriogram. Note superior mesenteric (SMV) and portal (PV) veins.

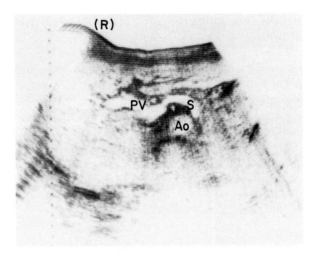

**Fig. 4-3.** Transverse scan showing splenic (S) and portal (PV) veins.

teric (SMV), and main portal (PV) veins. The splenic vein passes from the spleen toward the right. Just to the right of midline, it is joined by the superior mesenteric vein to become the portal vein.

On the transverse sonogram (Fig. 4-3), the splenic vein (S) is a very sonolucent structure which passes over the SMA and becomes enlarged as it courses to the right. This bulbous area represents the confluence of the splenic and superior mesenteric veins as they join to become the main portal vein (PV). To the right, the main portal vein bifurcates into right and left branches.

*Aorta.* The aorta (Fig. 4-4, Ao) is seen as a relatively sonolucent structure just anterior to the spine or, perhaps, slightly to the left of the midline. Low level

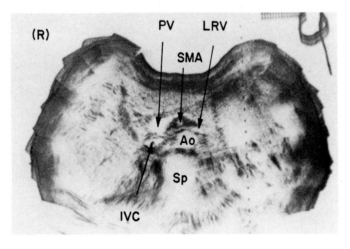

**Fig. 4-4.** Transverse scan.

echo activity is usually seen within the aorta, probably produced by turbulence of the red blood cells within.

*Superior mesenteric artery (SMA).*   The SMA is seen just anterior to the aorta and somewhat to the right. The splenic vein passes anterior to the SMA. Occasionally, one may visualize a vascular structure passing between the SMA and aorta. This structure represents the left renal vein (LRV) as it courses from the left kidney to the inferior vena cava.

*Inferior vena cava (IVC).*   The inferior vena cava has a very variable size and shape, but usually is elliptical and located adjacent and to the right of the aorta.

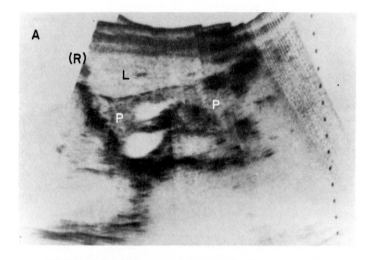

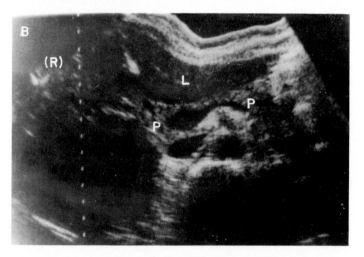

**Fig. 4-5.**   (A) Transverse scan—white background. The pancreas (P) is more echogenic than the liver (L). (B) Transverse scan—black background.

The location of the pancreas relative to these structures is demonstrated in Figs.4-5A and 4-5B. So that those used to either white or black backgrounds are not offended, both have been reproduced. The pancreas (P) is relatively echogenic —somewhat more so than the adjacent liver. The tail is that portion of the gland to the left of the aorta and SMA. The body lies in close proximity to the aorta and becomes the neck where the SMV joins the splenic vein to become the portal vein. Finally, the head lies just anterior to the inferior vena cava. As can be appreciated, the splenic vein is the most important landmark on the transverse scan and, indeed, was thought by many to represent the pancreas in the days before gray scale.

With respect to the pancreas, three longitudinal scans of the basic abdominal sonogram have been found to be of particular value:

1. Over the aorta and SMA. The body of the pancreas lies just anterior to these structures (Fig.4-6, arrows).
2. Over the SMV. The neck of the pancreas passes over this structure. (Fig. 7A, 7B). Frequently, the aorta and SMV lie in the same sagittal plane. It should be noted that the uncinate process of the pancreas lies posterior to the SMV. Embryologically, the uncinate process arises as a separate structure posterior to the head. During development, the uncinate process unites with the head, leaving the SMV between the head and neck of the pancreas anteriorly and the uncinate process posteriorly.
3. Over the inferior vena cava. The pancreatic head (P) lies just anterior to the IVC just caudal to the point where the IVC passes into or posterior to the liver (Fig. 4-8). Walls and Templeton have reported a number of cases in which pancreatic head masses have caused reproducible compression on the anterior aspect of the IVC.[2] Experience has shown that this portion of the inferior vena cava is very difficult to visualize because of the presence of gas.

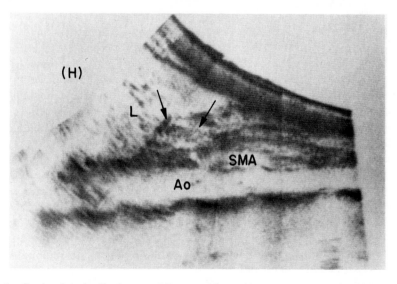

**Fig. 4-6.** Supine longitudinal scan. Note position of pancreas (arrows) with respect to aorta (Ao), SMA, and liver (L).

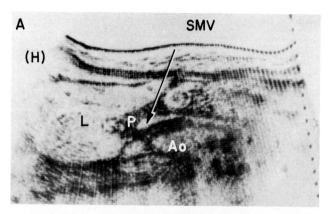

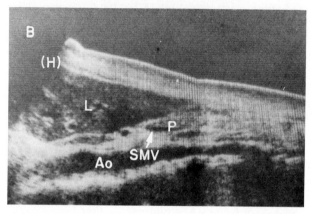

**Fig. 4-7 A and B.** White (A) and black (B) longitudinal scans. Note positions of SMV relative to the pancreas (P) and liver (L).

Simonds and associates have recently performed a statistical analysis on 100 normal people to determine the size of the pancreas.[3] The pancreatic head was found to measure approximately 2 cm on both the longitudinal and transverse sections, while the neck measured approximately 1 cm on both sections. The authors, however, claim that in addition to size, tissue consistency is an important factor in detecting pancreatic lesions.

We have not been impressed with the ultrasonic evaluation of the pancreatic tail. One may use the sonographic windows provided by the left kidney, spleen, and fluid-filled stomach, but these very limited windows and normal variations in the size and shape of the pancreatic tail make this an unreliable examination for the detection of edema or carcinoma. A recent paper by Simonds describes a technique whereby improved imaging of the pancreatic tail may be achieved.[4] The technique basically involves filling the stomach with water, waiting for the microbubbles to disperse and obtaining supine transverse scans of the left upper quadrant. The pancreatic tail can also be visualized in the prone position between the left kidney and the fluid-filled stomach.

Using this technique, more success has been demonstrated in attempts to visualize the pancreatic tail. In the longitudinal supine scan below (Fig. 4-9A), the

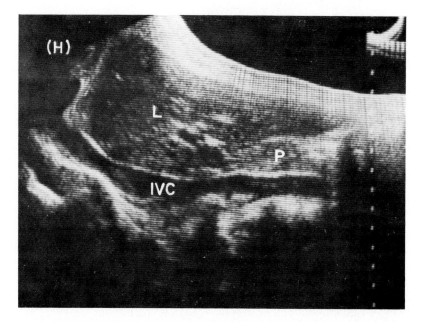

**Fig. 4-8.** Longitudinal scan. Note position of pancreas (P) relative to the IVC and liver (L).

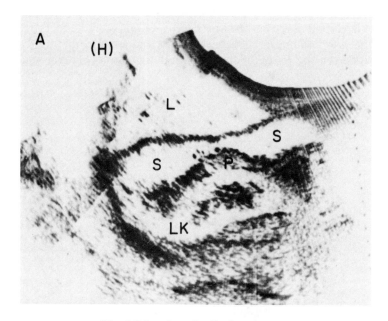

**Fig. 4-9 A.** Longitudinal supine scan.

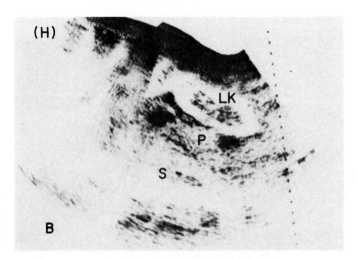

**Fig. 4-9 B.** Longitudinal prone scan.

pancreatic tail (P) is visualized just between the left kidney (LK) and fluid-filled stomach (S).

On the prone longitudinal scan (Fig. 4-9B), the pancreatic tail (P) is visualized between the left kidney (LK) and fluid-filled stomach (S).

Finally, no examination of the pancreas is complete without sonographic study of the biliary tree. Since cholecystitis is considered one of the conditions associated with pancreatitis, it is essential to rule out the presence of stones. Moreover, because of the close anatomic relation of the common bile duct to the pancreatic head, pathology in the latter can lead to profound effects in the biliary tree. As demonstrated in Fig. 4-9C below, the common bile duct (CBD) is essentially embedded in the tissue of the pancreatic head at its lateral and posterior margin.

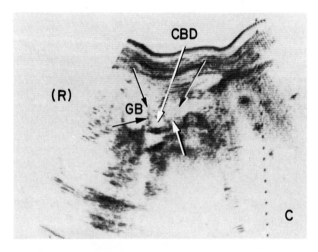

**Fig. 4-9 C.** Transverse scan. Note position of CBD relative to pancreas (arrows).

### Case

FC is a 32-year-old male who presented with severe epigastric pain. An upper GI series performed on two occasions revealed the presence of a constant impression on the medial aspect of the descending duodenum (Fig. 4-10, arrows). Representative longitudinal and transverse scans are shown below (Figs. 4-11, 4-12, 4-13).

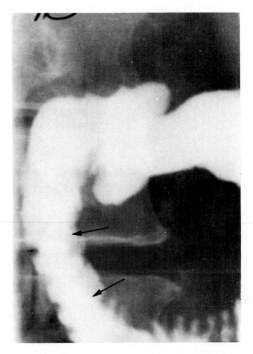

**Fig. 4-10.**   Spot film from upper GI series. There is an impression on the medial wall of the descending duodenum (arrow).

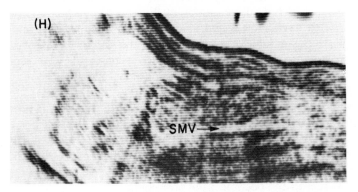

**Fig. 4-11.**   Longitudinal scan. The SMV is labeled.

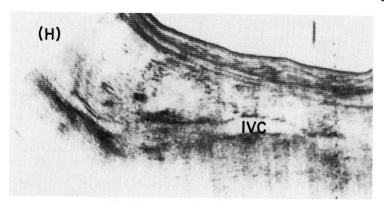

**Fig. 4-12.**   Longitudinal scan. The IVC is labeled.

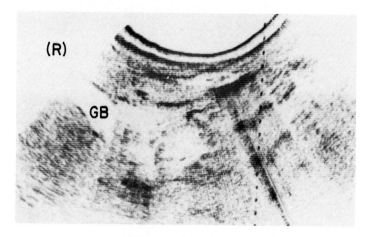

**Fig. 4-13.**   Transverse scan of epigastrium. The gallbladder is labeled.

DISCUSSION

On the transverse scan, the normal pancreatic head occupies a small corner of the anatomy in the right upper quadrant (Fig. 4-14A). Other structures, such as the inferior vena cava, portal and splenic veins, right kidney, and gallbladder present many acoustic interfaces which make the sonographic appearance quite complex. Now compare the normal transverse scan to the case reported above (Fig. 4-14B). There is a relatively homogeneous mass (M) which obscures much of the detailed anatomy seen in normal patients.

Compare the sagittal scan obtained over the SMV and IVC in normal patients (Figs. 4-15A and 4-16A to those obtained in the patient FC (Figs. 4-15B, 4-16B). The space occupied by normal pancreatic tissue is quite small, usually measuring less than 2 cm in depth, and in some patients hardly visualized at all. In FC, the amount of pancreatic tissue visualized adjacent to the SMV and IVC (Fig. 4-15B, 4-16B) has increased and become quite prominent.

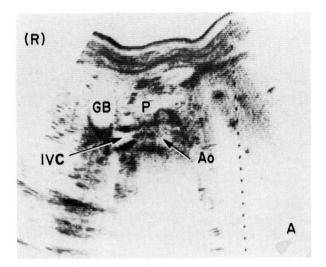

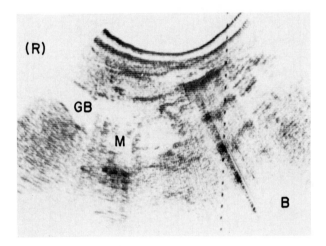

**Fig. 4-14.** (A) Transverse scan in patient with slightly dilated gallbladder and CBD. Note sharp acoustic interfaces caused by the various structures in the epigastrium. (B) Transverse scan in patient FC. The normal structures are obliterated by the relatively sonolucent mass (M).

Again, referring to the normal and abnormal scans reproduced, compare the echogenic activity of the normal pancreas and that of the edematous pancreas. As mentioned in the introduction to this chapter, normal pancreatic tissue is quite echogenic, generally more so than the liver. In acute pancreatitis, the gland becomes edematous and considerably less echogenic than the adjacent liver. The edematous gland also attenuates less sound and greater through transmission is apparent as compared to the normal gland. Portions of the pancreas may be so sonolucent that one may suspect the presence of a small area of fluid accumulation or pseudocyst.

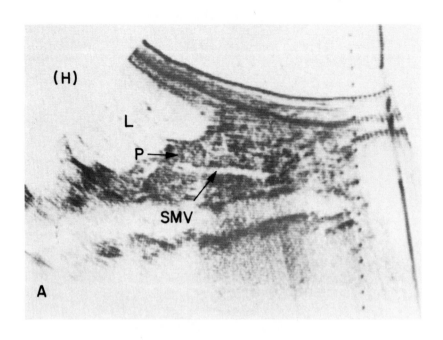

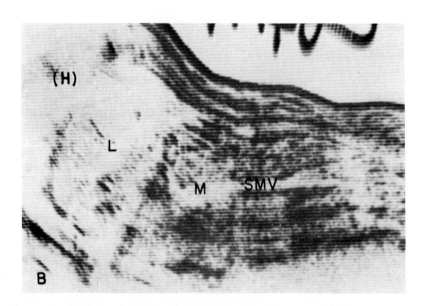

**Fig. 4-15.** (A) Longitudinal scan of SMV in normal patient. (B) Longitudinal scan of SMV in FC. Note relatively sonolucent mass (M) in area of pancreatic neck.

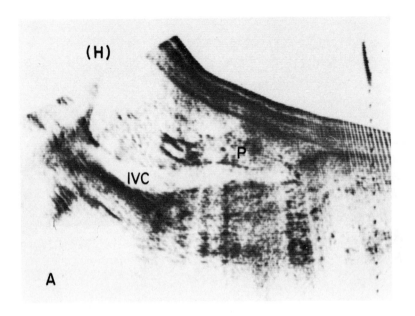

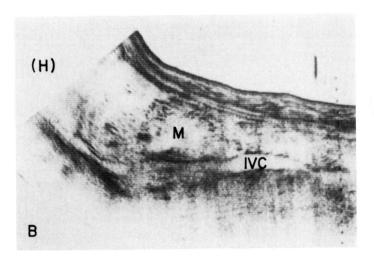

**Fig. 4-16.** (A) Longitudinal scan of IVC in normal patient. (B) Longitudinal scan of IVC in FC. Again, note mass (M) anterior to the IVC.

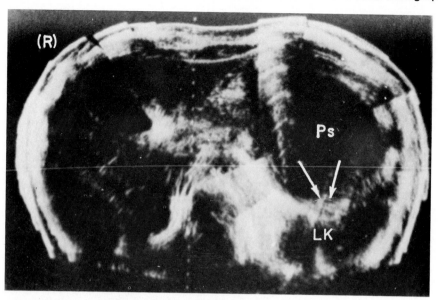

**Fig. 4-17.** Transverse scan showing large pseudocyst (Ps) of the pancreatic tail just anterior to the left kidney (LK). Note debris within the pseudocyst (arrows).

FOLLOW UP

The patient, lost to follow up for approximately eight months, finally returned, and a sonographic examination was performed (Fig. 4-17). A large cystic structure with debris (arrows) was identified, which was proven at surgery to represent a pancreatic pseudocyst.

COMMENTS

1. Acute pancreatitis has been found to be a somewhat difficult diagnosis to make. As a response to the disease process itself, these patients frequently have considerable gas in their gastrointestinal tracts. Consequently, much of the sonographic window into the upper abdomen, which is so critical for evaluation of the pancreas is lost. As mentioned previously, angling the transducer approximately 10 degrees toward the feet may eliminate some of these problems.
2. Needless to say, pseudocyst formation is a common sequela of pancreatitis. Pseudocysts can be very variable in their location and careful search of the abdomen, including the left upper quadrant, should be considered part of a routine sonogram.

### Case

JS is a 78-year-old male admitted with dull epigastric pain and weight loss. Portions of his sonographic study are shown below (Figs. 4-18, 4-19, 4-20, 4-21). What portions of the biliary tree are dilated? Are you secure in making a diagnosis or would you recommend further studies?

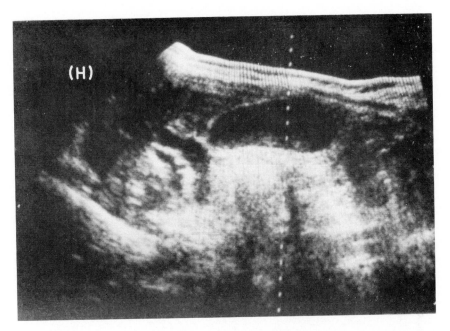

**Fig. 4-18.** Longitudinal scan.

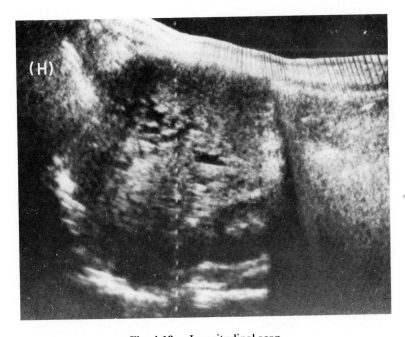

**Fig. 4-19.** Longitudinal scan.

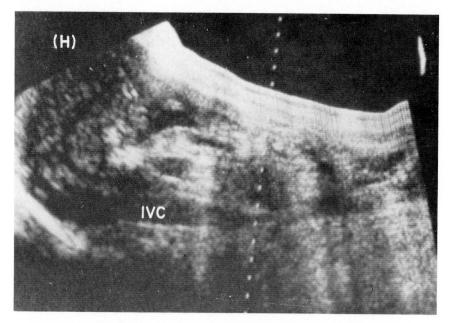

**Fig. 4-20.** Longitudinal scan. The IVC is labeled.

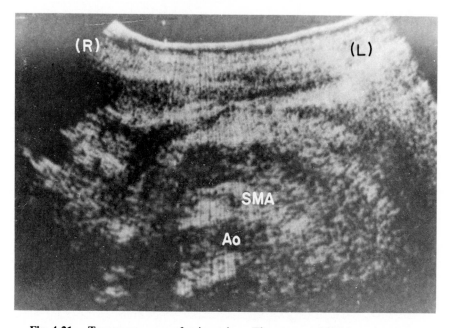

**Fig. 4-21.** Transverse scan of epigastrium. The aorta and SMA are labeled.

DISCUSSION

Fig. 4-22 reveals a markedly dilated gallbladder and dilated common bile duct (CBD). Following a fatty meal, the gallbladder did not contract significantly. The biliary radicles are also dilated (Fig. 4-23, arrows).

In Fig. 4-24A, the etiology behind the distention of the biliary tree can begin to be appreciated. A mass (M) is identified anterior to the IVC. Compare Fig. 4-24A to the normal longitudinal section of the IVC (Fig. 4-24B).

Finally, the transverse scan reveals a relatively homogeneous mass (M) in the

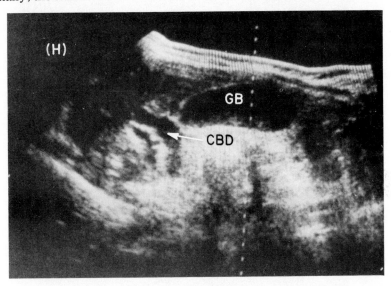

**Fig. 4-22.** Longitudinal scan. Note dilated gallbladder and CBD.

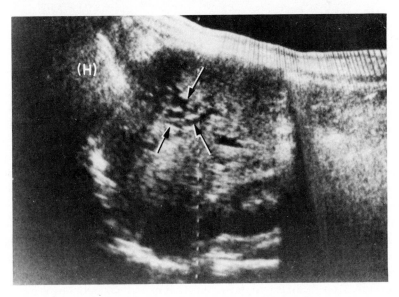

**Fig. 4-23.** Longitudinal scan. Note dilated bile ducts (arrows).

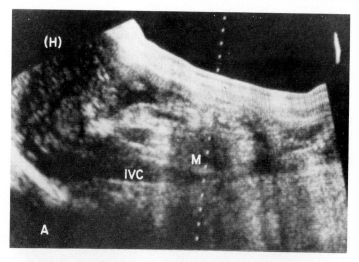

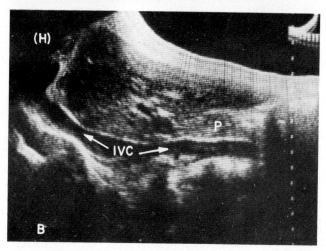

**Fig. 4-24.** (A) Longitudinal scan showing mass (M) over IVC. (B) Longitudinal scan over IVC in normal patient.

area of the pancreatic neck and head (Fig. 4-25A). A transverse scan of the epigastrium in another patient with carcinoma of the pancreatic head is shown in Fig. 4-27B. A normal transverse scan is reproduced for comparison (Fig. 4-25C).

FOLLOW UP

A transhepatic cholangiogram revealed tapering of the distal common bile duct, suggestive of neoplastic involvement. At surgery, carcinoma of the pancreatic head with involvement of the uncinate process was identified.

COMMENTS

1.  Returning to the classification of dilated gallbladders considered in Chapter 3 it can be seen that this case falls into category III. As mentioned concerning acute pancreatitis, carcinoma of the pancreas is also a difficult sonographic diagnosis. It has been found, however, that pancreatic neoplasms have a more discrete appearance than edematous portions of the pancreas. As one would expect, pancreatic edema tends to be more diffuse, frequently involving the

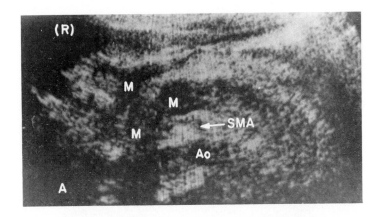

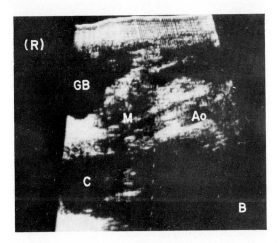

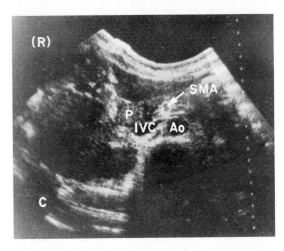

**Fig. 4-25.** (A) Transverse scan of epigastrium. Note mass (M). (B) Transverse scan of epigastrium in another patient with a mass (M) involving the head and neck of the pancreas. This patient had a dilated gallbladder (GB) and right renal cyst (C). (C) Transverse scan of epigastrium in a normal patient.

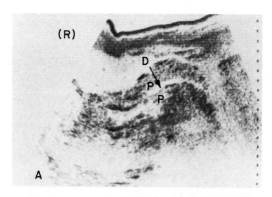

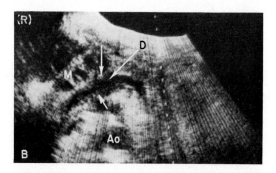

**Fig. 4-26.** (A) Transverse scan of epigastrium. Note pancreatic duct (D) within pancreatic tissue (P). (B) Transverse scan of epigastrium. Note pancreatic duct (D) surrounded by pancreatic tissue (arrows). The mass (M) has a lobulated appearance in this patient.

entire gland. Carcinoma, on the other hand, generally involves a localized portion of the gland. Of course, if neoplastic involvement is advanced, a large portion of the gland may be affected.

In terms of tissue characterization, neoplasm often presents a more echogenic appearance than does pancreatic edema. There is also more tissue attenuation through neoplastic lesions with consequently less through transmission than with edematous portions of the gland.

When dealing with the pancreatic head, there is frequently another clue that enables one to distinguish between inflammatory disease and neoplasm—obstruction of the common bile duct. Although chronic inflammatory disease of the pancreas has been reported to cause obstruction of the common bile duct, carcinoma of the pancreas is a far more common cause. It is safe to say that when a pancreatic mass is discovered in combination with a dilated biliary tree or gallbladder, carcinoma of the pancreas should be considered until proven otherwise. As mentioned previously, early in the disease the gallbladder may be the only portion of the biliary tree to dilate appreciably.

Finally, the discrimination between carcinoma and pancreatitis is aided enormously by the clinical history. Although, surely borderline cases do exist, the clinical stories are usually very different.

2. Gosink and Leopold have reported a sonographic sign that suggests obstructive disease near the ampulla of Vater.[5] When there is longstanding obstruc-

tion at this level, not only does the biliary tree dilate, but the pancreatic duct may dilate as well. In the transverse scan opposite (Fig. 4-26A), one may appreciate a sonolucent structure (D) in the middle of the pancreatic tissue. This patient did have carcinoma of the pancreatic head and neck with obstruction of the common bile duct near the ampulla of Vater. A transverse scan (Fig. 4-26B) in another patient is reproduced as well. Again, a sonolucent structure (D) is identified within the midst of the pancreatic tissue (arrows). The mass (M) in this case has a very lobulated appearance, and at surgery turned out to be metastatic adenopathy within the *porta hepatis*. The common bile duct was obstructed at the ampulla.

### Case

NT is a 52-year-old female referred to our department for a gallbladder sonogram. For approximately one year prior to admission, she had experienced vague upper abdominal discomfort during and after meals. The patient claimed to have lost approximately 30 pounds since the onset of these symptoms. Her first imaging examination was a gallbladder sonogram. No gallstones were found, but the routine abdominal sonogram which served as the basis of our gallbladder study produced unexpected results. Below are supine longitudinal and transverse scans (Fig. 4-27, 4-28).

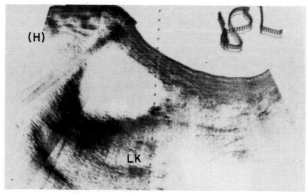

**Fig. 4-27.** Supine longitudinal scan of the left upper quadrant. The left kidney (LK) is labeled.

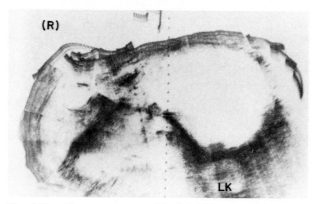

**Fig. 4-28.** Transverse scan. The left kidney (LK) is labeled.

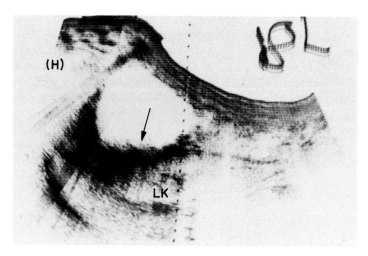

**Fig. 4-29.** Supine longitudinal scan of the left upper quadrant. Note debris within the cyst (arrow).

DISCUSSION

The supine longitudinal and transverse scans (Fig. 4-29, 4-30) reveal a sonolucent mass in the left upper quadrant which appears to be just anterior to the left kidney (LK). Debris is seen within the cyst (arrows).

Prone and decubitus longitudinal scanning of the left upper quadrant is quite helpful in evaluating pancreatic tail lesions. Using the left kidney and spleen as sonographic windows, the posterior aspect of the mass adjacent to the left kidney may be better visualized. Fig. 4-31 below is an example of a prone scan. The pseudocyst (PS) and its relation to the left kidney can be appreciated. The cyst is adjacent to, but does not deform the left renal outline.

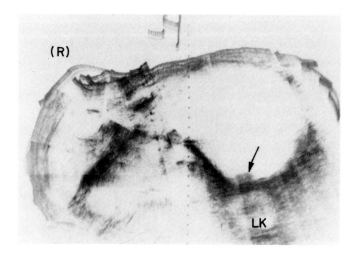

**Fig. 4-30.** Transverse scan.

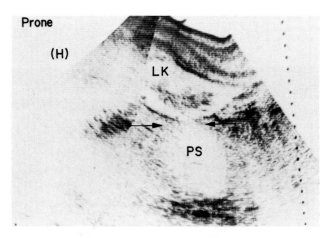

**Fig. 4-31.** Prone longitudinal scan. Note relationship of cyst (Ps) to kidney.

FOLLOW UP

An upper GI series revealed a large, extragastric mass associated with a very prominent impression on the stomach (Fig. 4-32). At surgery, a pancreatic pseudocyst was found.

COMMENTS

1. At the risk of becoming repetitious, one must again point out the importance of performing a basic abdominal sonogram as part of the gallbladder, pancreatic, or liver study. The clinician of the patient reported above was suspicious that gallstones were responsible for the symptoms. We were unable to find any evidence of cholelithiasis but managed to find the cause of the pa-

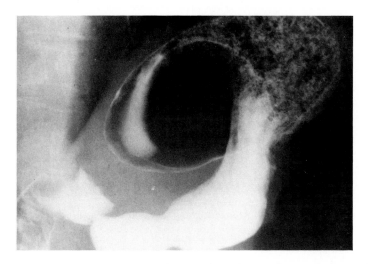

**Fig. 4-32.** Upper GI series showing prominent impression on the stomach.

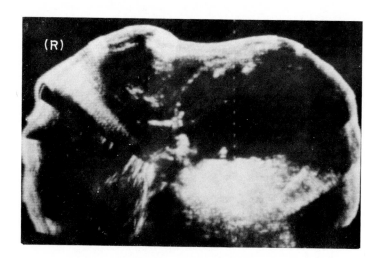

**Fig. 4-33.**   Transverse scan.

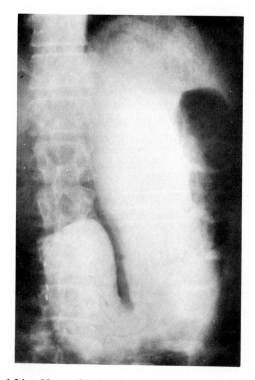

**Fig. 4-34.**   Upper GI showing markedly dilated stomach.

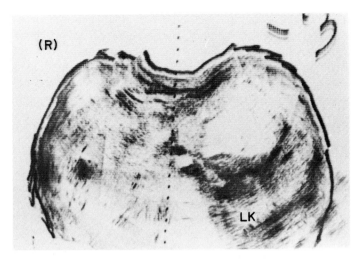

**Fig. 4-35.** Supine transverse scan. Note thick-walled cystic structure anterior to the left kidney.

tient's symptomatology. Following the appropriate therapy, the patient improved dramatically.

2. Opposite is a transverse section of the upper abdomen in a patient with severe nausea, vomiting, and left upper quadrant discomfort (Fig. 4-33). Admittedly, the scan is of suboptimal technique because of the patient's unstable clinical condition. Are we again dealing with a large pseudocyst?

An upper GI series revealed a markedly dilated stomach (Fig. 4-34) filled with fluid and debris. This pitfall can be avoided by visualizing the dilated stomach on a KUB or upper GI series.

Fig. 4-35 is a scan on another patient with a sonolucent left upper quadrant mass. The mass is just anterior to the left kidney and has thickened walls. The preoperative diagnosis of a mature pseudocyst was made, but was incorrect. At surgery, an acinar cell carcinoma of the pancreatic tail was encountered.

Splenic pathology, such as cysts, may also present as sonolucent masses in the left upper quadrant. The reader is referred to Taylor's very complete description of the ultrasonic characteristics of the spleen and its pathology in *Atlas of Gray Scale Ultrasonography*.[6]

SUMMARY

The basic abdominal sonogram described in Chapter 1 serves as the backbone of the pancreatic sonogram. The modifications of the basic procedure include careful single-sweep sectoring of the epigastrium in the transverse plane. The problems caused by bowel gas may, to some extent, be eliminated by angling the transducer approximately 10 degrees toward the feet. Important longitudinal scans include sections over the aorta and SMA, SMV, and IVC.

Acute pancreatitis generally presents as diffuse, homogeneous enlargement of the pancreas. Instead of being more echogenic then the adjacent liver, the edematous pancreas presents as a relatively sonolucent mass with appreciable through transmission. Carcinoma, on the other hand, is generally more echogenic and discrete. Involvement of the biliary tree serves as an important clue of underlying pancreatic head neoplasm. Pancreatic pseudocysts present as sonolucent structures, many of which have debris within. Pseudocysts must be distinguished from other causes of sonolucent abdominal masses, such as the fluid-filled obstructed stomach, left renal cysts, and splenic cysts.

**REFERENCES**

1.  Filly RA, Goldberg BB: Normal vessels, in Goldberg BB (ed): Abdominal Gray Scale Ultrasonography. New York, Wiley, 1977, p 19
2.  Walls W, Templeton A: The ultrasonic demonstration of inferior vena caval compression: A guide to pancreatic head enlargement with emphasis on neoplasm. Radiology 123:165–167, 1977
3.  Simonds BD, Taylor KJW, Rosenfield AT, et al: Gray-scale echography of the pancreas: Re-evaluation of normal size. Radiology (in press)
4.  Simonds BD: Normal anatomy of the pancreas. Ultrasound Clinics (in press)
5.  Gosink BB, Leopold GR: The dilated pancreatic duct: Ultrasonic evaluation. Radiology 126:477–478, 1978
6.  Taylor KJW: Atlas of gray scale ultrasonography. New York, Churchill Livingstone, 1978, p 170

# 5

# The Liver

As a result of its position and sonographic characteristics, the liver is an excellent organ to evaluate by means of ultrasound. Examination of its biliary system has been discussed in Chapters 2 and 3. The normal liver parenchyma presents a fine homogeneous echo pattern (Fig. 5-1). Moreover, the majority of this organ can be scanned without the impediments of ribs and gas. As of this writing, however, the value of liver sonography in the overall workup of liver disease has not been completely resolved. Radionuclide sulfur colloid and gallium studies of the liver are, of course, the alternative examinations. CT scanning, although not as widely used, has also proved to be valuable in detecting liver lesions.[1,2]

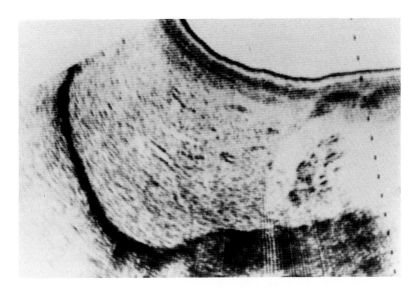

**Fig. 5-1.** Longitudinal scan. Note fine homogeneous echo pattern of the liver.

**INDICATIONS**

1.  Evaluation of fluid-filled structures, such as abscesses and cysts within the liver. Because of the echogenicity of the surrounding normal liver parenchyma, fluid-filled masses are clearly defined.
2.  Evaluation of fluid collections around the liver, such as subphrenic abscesses and ascites.
3.  Evaluation of diffuse hepatocellular disease, such as cirrhosis. This indication has somewhat limited use at the present time, but will probably become more important with the advent of digital scan converters.
4.  Evaluation of right upper quadrant masses.
5.  As a complement to the sulfur colloid liver scan. At present, the sulfur colloid liver scan remains a basic screening procedure at the vast majority of institutions. On a good isotope scan, the entire outline of the liver can be seen in several different views. This is not the case with the sector scanner by which only small slices of the liver are visualized with each pass. Real time systems have significant advantage in such a large organ as the liver.

   Since the sulfur colloid liver scan is the most widespread screening examination of the liver, let us consider the various results of this study that may lead us to perform a liver sonogram as a complementary procedure.

   *Abnormal liver scan.* Certainly, there are cases in which a sulfur colloid scan is so positive in patients with a known primary neoplasm, that further investigation would be unnecessary. Below, is a typical example (Fig. 5-2). The patient

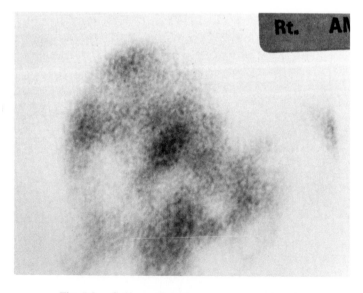

**Fig. 5-2.** Sulfur colloid liver scan—anterior view.

had carcinoma of the lung with a very positive sulfur colloid liver scan. Unless the course of treatments were followed, a liver sonogram would be redundant. There are many cases, however, when a liver sonogram could better characterize focal areas of diminished activity on the sulfur colloid scan. The enlarged gallbladder bed (see p. 42) is a typical example.

*Equivocal liver scan.*  By definition, the equivocal liver scan is not clearly positive or negative, and sonography serves as an excellent complementary procedure.

*Normal liver scan.*  The sulfur colloid scan is relatively insensitive in the detection of early metastatic lesions. Ultrasound, used as a complementary procedure, can substantially increase the sensitivity. Taylor, in fact, claims that ultrasound is more sensitive in detecting early metastatic lesions.[3] Experience will depend on how sophisticated and well adjusted one's equipment is and how compulsively one does one's liver sonography.

## TECHNIQUE

The basic abdominal sonogram described in Chapter 1 provides the backbone of the liver sonogram. The transverse sections provide the gross anatomic information, while the longitudinal views are useful in the evaluation of subtle changes in the parenchymal architecture. As mentioned in Chapter 1, the longitudinal scans begin just to the left of midline over the left lobe of the liver, and proceed at 1 cm intervals toward the right until further scanning is prevented by the right costal margin. Additional oblique views of the liver can be obtained by scanning perpendicular to the right costal margin.

According to the technique advocated by Taylor, the TGC, or Time-Gain Compensation curve, should be adjusted so that the amplitude of the intrahepatic echoes are approximately the same throughout the depth of the liver.[4] The amplitude of these low-level echoes should be between one-third and one-half the amplitude of the diaphragmatic echoes.

### Case

RK is a 48-year-old female admitted with fever, elevated white blood count, and right upper quadrant pain. The patient's clinician was suspicious of cholecystitis and ordered a gallbladder sonogram. Supine longitudinal and transverse sonograms are shown below (Fig. 5-3, 5-4, 5-5, 5-6). Pay particular attention to where the scans were obtained. Fig. 5-3 is a transverse section approximately 3 cm from the xyphoid, while Fig. 5-4 is approximately 8 cm below the xyphoid. Fig. 5-5 is a supine longitudinal scan 3 cm to the right of midline and, finally, Fig. 5-6 is 5 cm to the right of midline. Can you appreciate two distinct sonolucent masses?

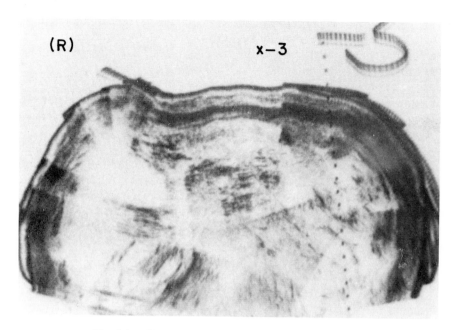

**Fig. 5-3.** Transverse scan—3 cm below the xyphoid.

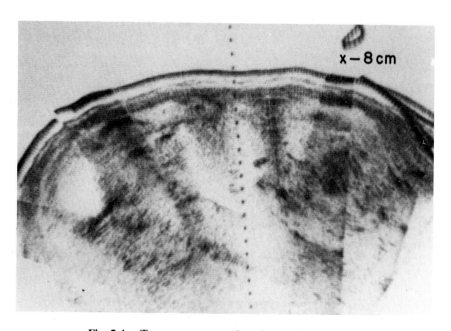

**Fig. 5-4.** Transverse scan—8 cm below the xyphoid.

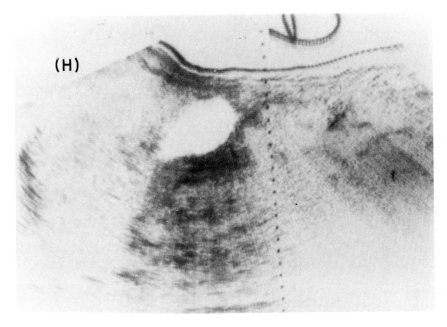

**Fig. 5-5.** Supine longitudinal scan—3 cm to the right of midline.

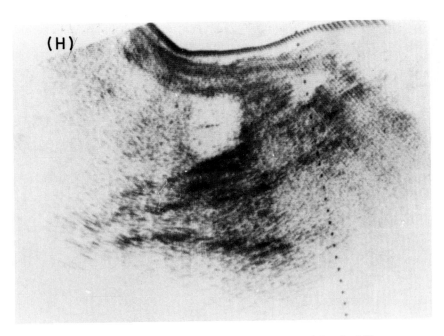

**Fig. 5-6.** Supine longitudinal scan—5 cm to the right of midline.

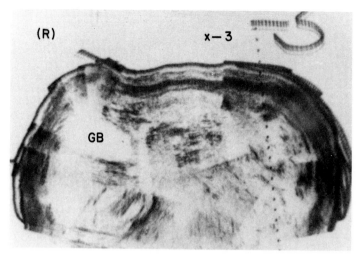

**Fig. 5-7.** Transverse scan—3 cm below the xyphoid. Note the dilated gallbladder.

DISCUSSION

Fig.5-7 and 5-8 reveal a slightly dilated gallbladder where one would expect to find the gallbladder.

Fig. 5-9 is a transverse section taken approximately 5 cm from the scan in Fig. 5-7. Note another separate sonolucent mass (M) below and lateral to the gallbladder. Figure 5-10 is a longitudinal section lateral to the gallbladder and again reveals a relatively sonolucent mass (M) at the tip of the liver. A linear interface (arrow) is noted within the sonolucent mass, probably representing a fluid level.

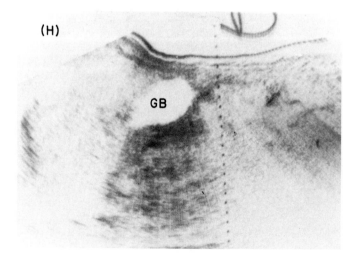

**Fig. 5-8.** Supine longitudinal scan—3 cm to the right of midline. Note dilated gallbladder.

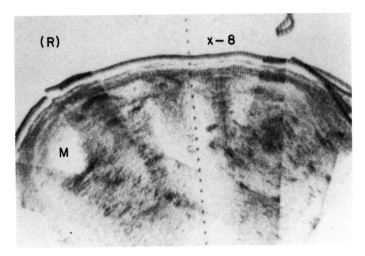

**Fig. 5-9.** Transverse scan—8 cm below the xyphoid. Note fluid collection on the right (M).

FOLLOW UP

A gallium scan revealed concentration of the isotope in the right upper quadrant after 48 hours (Fig. 5-11). The patient was treated with antibiotics, recovered, and was discharged before a repeat examination could be performed.

COMMENT

This case, and another like it (Fig. 5-12, 5-13), are deceptive. To the unwary, the abscesses (Ab) at the tip of the liver (L) may be mistaken for a dilated gallbladder.

A similar picture may be obtained when ascitic fluid surrounds the tip of the

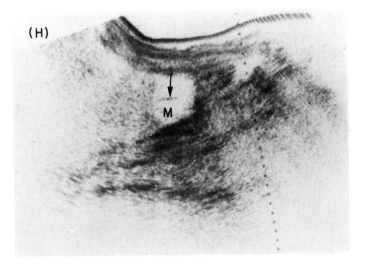

**Fig. 5-10.** Supine longitudinal scan—5 cm to the right of midline. Note the relatively sonolucent mass (M) with fluid level (arrows).

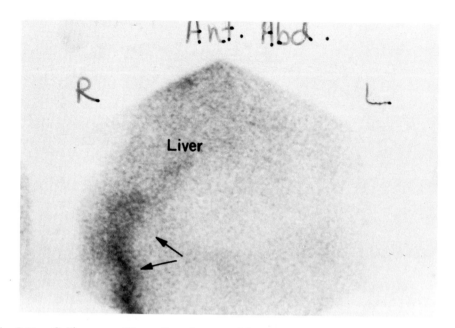

**Fig. 5-11.** Gallium scan. The radioactive material concentrates just below the liver at the end of 48 hours.

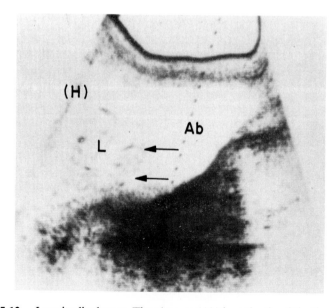

**Fig. 5-12.** Longitudinal scan. The abscess (Ab) is at the tip of the liver (L).

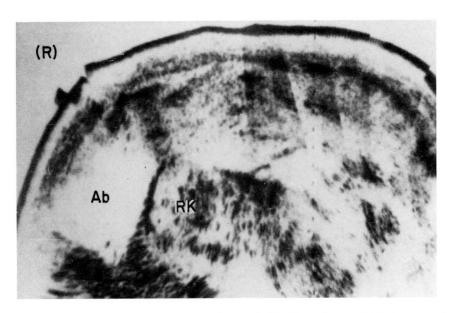

**Fig. 5-13.** Transverse scan—8 cm below the xyphoid. The abscess (Ab) is just lateral to the right kidney (RK).

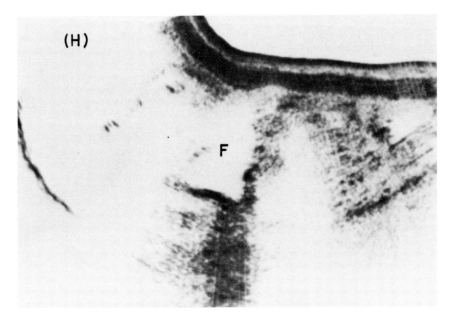

**Fig. 5-14.** Longitudinal scan. There is ascitic fluid (F) at the tip of the liver.

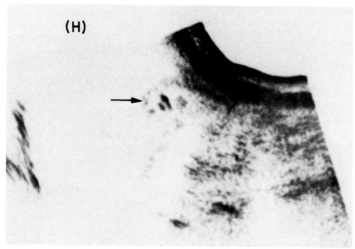

**Fig. 5-15.** Longitudinal scan. The sonolucent mass (M) is again present. Note small gallbladder with stone (arrow).

liver on longitudinal scan. In the longitudinal scan (Fig. 5-14), the fluid (F) around the edge of the liver has an appearance not unlike a dilated gallbladder or abscess. The gallbladder, however, is more cephalad in location (Fig. 5-15, arrow). Incidentally, there is a stone in this gallbladder.

### Cases A and B

Below are supine longitudinal scans in two different patients (Fig. 5-16, 5-17). Where are the fluid collections?

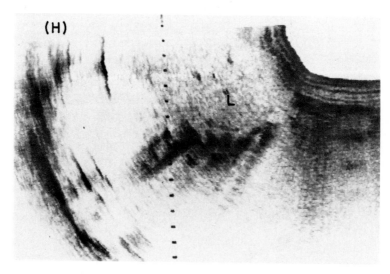

**Fig. 5-16.** Case A, supine longitudinal scan. The liver (L) is labeled. (Courtesy of Dr. Steven Gerzof, Boston Veterans Hospital).

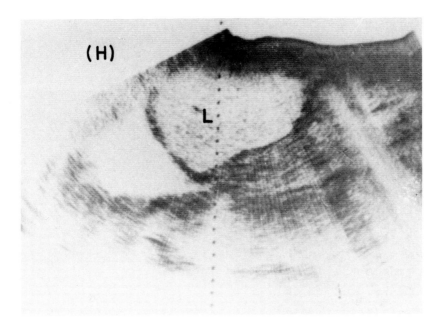

**Fig. 5-17.** Case B, longitudinal scan. The liver is labeled.

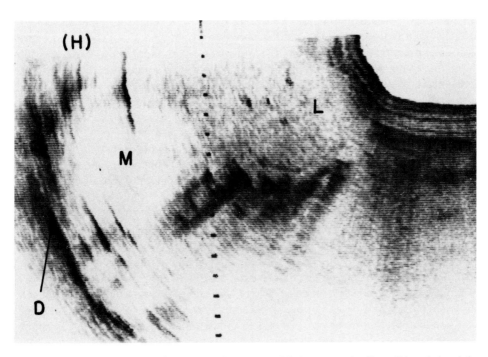

**Fig. 5-18.** Case A, longitudinal scan. Note mass (M) between the liver (L) and the right hemidiaphragm (D).

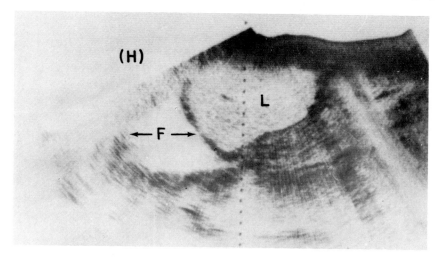

**Fig. 5-19.** Case B, longitudinal scan. Fluid (F) is noted between the right hemidiaphragm and right lung (arrows).

DISCUSSION

In Case A (Fig. 5-18) there is a relatively sonolucent mass (M) between the liver and the right hemidiaphragm. Therefore, the fluid is subphrenic in location. Incidentally, the shadowing within the liver itself is caused by surgical clips.

In Case B (Fig. 5-19) the fluid is above the right hemidiaphragm and represents right pleural effusion. Ordinarily, normal air-containing lung above the right hemidiaphragm acts as a barrier to the transmission of sound (Fig. 5-20). But the presence of pleural fluid allows the transmission of sound some distance above the diaphragm (Fig. 5-19, arrows).

FOLLOW UP

Case A—A radionuclide liver-lung scan revealed significant separation of the dome of the liver from the base of the right lung. Following percutaneous drainage of the subphrenic abscess, the patient improved dramatically (See comments, p. 108).

Case B—The patient had congestive heart failure with right pleural effusion, which disappeared following appropriate therapy.

COMMENTS

1. Certainly, the use of ultrasound to establish the presence of pleural effusion is not advocated. Except in cases where the fluid may be loculated, the chest x-ray remains the examination of choice. Sonographic evaluation of the right hemidiaphragm, however, provides a quick and effective means of establishing the presence of a subphrenic fluid collection. In addition, the excursion of the right hemidiaphragm can be determined by scanning the patient in full inspiration and then, on the same scan, in full expiration (Fig. 5-21). This

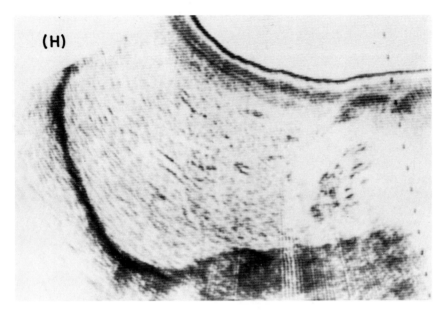

**Fig. 5-20.** Longitudinal scan. Normal patient.

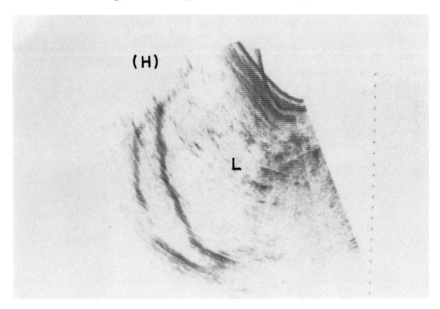

**Fig. 5-21.** Longitudinal scan. Both inspiratory and expiratory positions of the right hemi-diaphragm are included in the same scan.

procedure can also be performed on the left side by using the spleen and left kidney as the acoustic windows.

2.  Gerzof and associates have developed a technique of percutaneously draining subphrenic abscesses.[5] Although other modalities are used, such as CT and x-ray, the technique relies mainly on ultrasonic guidance. After a safe window is determined, a catheter is directed under ultrasonic guidance into the abscess.

### Case

GG is a 57-year-old female admitted with jaundice and increasing abdominal girth. Longitudinal and transverse views of the right upper quadrant are shown below (Fig. 5-22, 5-23). Can the patient's admitting signs and symptoms be explained by these scans?

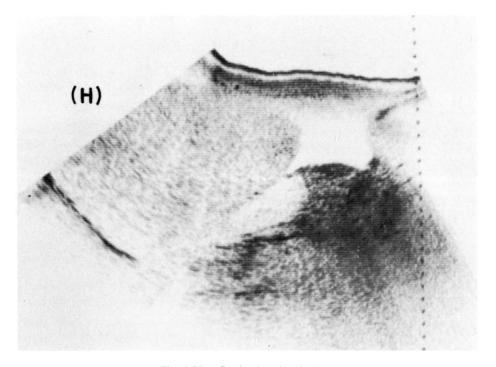

**Fig. 5-22.**  Supine longitudinal scan.

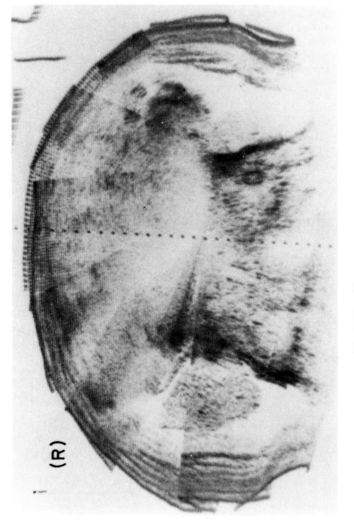

(R)

**Fig. 5-23.** Transverse scan.

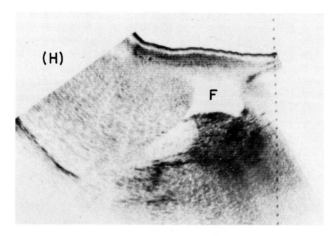

**Fig. 5-24.**   Supine longitudinal scan. Ascitic fluid (F) is noted at the tip of the liver.

DISCUSSION

These scans reveal the presence of fluid around the tip of the liver (Fig. 5-24, F) and around the flanks (Fig. 5-25, F). This fluid, of course, represents ascites.

In addition, the longitudinal scan of the liver (Fig. 5-26) reveals increased echo activity within the liver; the more superficial portions of the liver attenuate so much sound that the deeper portions appear relatively sonolucent. A normal liver scan is reproduced for comparison (Fig. 5-27). There was no evidence of a dilated biliary tree.

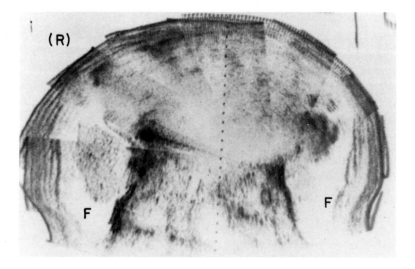

**Fig. 5-25.**   Transverse scan. Ascitic fluid (F) is noted around the root of the mesentery.

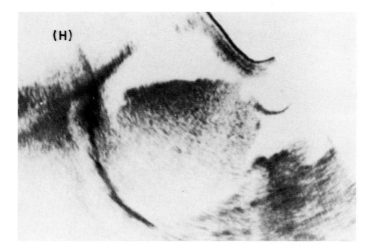

**Fig. 5-26.** Supine longitudinal scan. Note increased echo activity within the superficial portions of the liver.

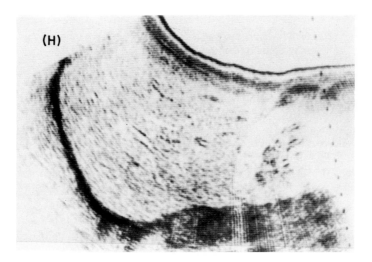

**Fig. 5-27.** Longitudinal scan. Normal liver parenchyma.

FOLLOW UP

A liver biopsy revealed the presence of diffuse hepatocellular disease with fibrosis compatible with cirrhosis.

COMMENTS

1.  Ultrasound provides an effective means of determining the presence of minimal ascites. This is another area where real time imaging has advantages over sector scanning. In the case reported above, the liver could actually be seen

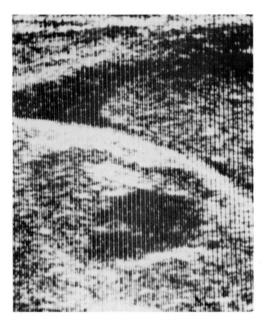

**Fig. 5-28.** Transverse scan. Part of a real time examination. Note the right renal cyst.

floating in the ascitic fluid. A transverse scan from the real time examination is shown below(Fig. 5-28).* Yes, a right renal cyst is present.
2.   Taylor has described the parenchyma of the cirrhotic liver as more echogenic than its normal counterpart.[6] As a result of increased attenuation of sound, the deeper portions of the liver appear relatively sonolucent. The constellation of findings above (increased echo activity within the liver parenchyma, no evidence of a dilated biliary tree, and ascites) is nearly diagnostic of jaundice caused by hepatocellular, rather than obstructive, disease.

### Cases A–E

HA is a 52-year-old female admitted with right upper quadrant pain. A gallbladder sonogram was ordered. Two representative longitudinal scans (Figs. 5-29, 5-30) are reproduced below. How much pathology can you identify?

*Study performed with a Toshiba Sonolayergraph sal-10A.

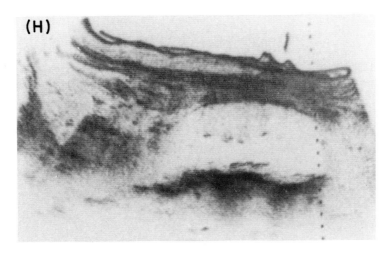

**Fig. 5-29.** Longitudinal scan at midline.

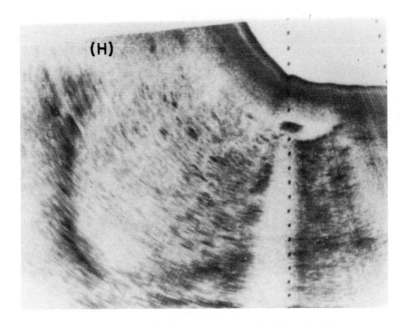

**Fig. 5-30.** Longitudinal scan at 3 cm to the right of midline.

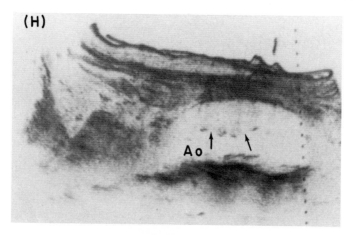

**Fig. 5-31.** Longitudinal scan showing abdominal aortic aneurysm with clot (arrows).

DISCUSSION

The longitudinal scan (Fig. 5-31) reveals an abdominal aortic aneurysm with clot formation (arrows). The longitudinal scan (Fig. 5-32) reveals a gallstone and abnormal liver parenchymal pattern. There are several well-circumscribed bulls-eye lesions, one of which is just cephalad to the shadow cast by the gallstone (arrows). Within the sonolucent rim of the lesion, there is tissue slightly more echogenic than the surrounding liver parenchyma.

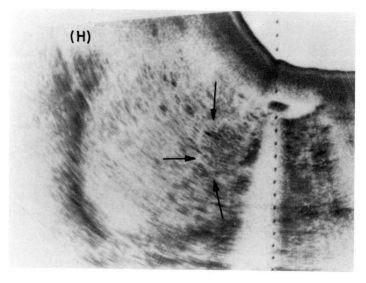

**Fig. 5-32.** Longitudinal scan. Note gallstone and bulls-eye lesion (arrows). There are other similar lesions present.

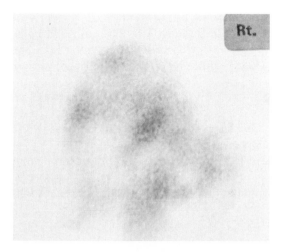

**Fig. 5-33.** Sulfur colloid liver scan—anterior view.

FOLLOW UP

The sulfur colloid liver scan (Fig. 5-33) reveals multiple focal defects compatible with metastatic disease. A barium enema performed subsequently revealed carcinoma of the sigmoid colon.

COMMENT

Several recent papers have been devoted to the description of metastatic lesions in the liver.[7-11] Our experience has been similar to that of Scheible, Gosink, and Leopold, who have classified liver metastasis into four categories—dense, lucent, bulls-eye, and other.[10] The case above falls into the category that is described as bulls-eye lesions. The metastatic focus (Fig. 5-34) is somewhat more

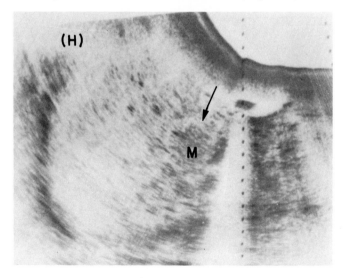

**Fig. 5-34.** Longitudinal scan—bulls-eye lesion.

echogenic than the surrounding liver parenchyma. A clearly defined rim of sono-lucent tissue surrounds a lesion (arrows). The so-called bulls-eye lesion can be deceiving. Occasionally, segments of hepatic veins can subtend sections of the liver parenchyma (Fig. 5-35A, 5-35B), resulting in a very similar sonographic appearance. As compared to the lucent rim around metastatic lesions, veins are usually quite straight and, if followed carefully, their branching pattern can be identified.

Case B is an example of multiple lucent metastases (Fig. 5-36, arrows). The larger lesion was palpable.

The diffuse pattern of Case C (Fig. 5-37) represents multiple, small sonolu-cent lesions.

Case D is an example of a dense, metastatic lesion. A longitudinal section is

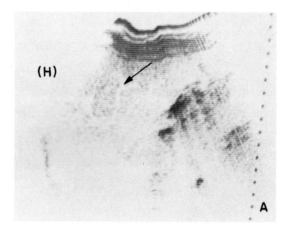

**Fig. 5-35 A.**   Longitudinal scan. Hepatic veins resulting in an appearance similar to bulls-eye lesions.

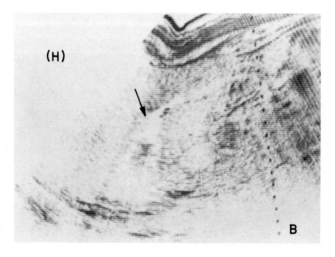

**Fig. 5-35 B.**   Horizontal scan. Hepatic vein is now clearly seen (arrow).

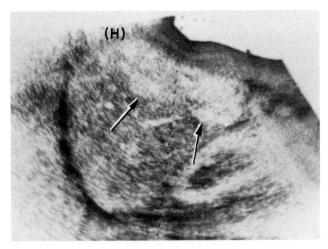

**Fig. 5-36.** Longitudinal scan. Multiple "lucent" metastasis (arrows).

shown in Fig. 5-38. A film from the upper GI series (Fig.5-39) is also shown. What is the primary?

The lesion in the duodenal bulb was a carcinoid and the large lesion in the liver was a metastasis. The radionuclide scan is reproduced in Fig. 5-40.

Finally, Case E is a 54-year-old female admitted with a three-month history of constipation. A barium enema (Fig. 5-41) revealed a neoplasm involving the descending portion of the large bowel. A radionuclide sulfur colloid scan (Fig. 5-42) revealed a focal defect within the liver at the junction of the right and left lobes (arrow).

These two findings considered together are very suggestive of metastatic carcinoma to the liver. A liver sonogram (Fig. 5-43), however, revealed a completely sonolucent lesion in the same area as the defect on the liver scan. The

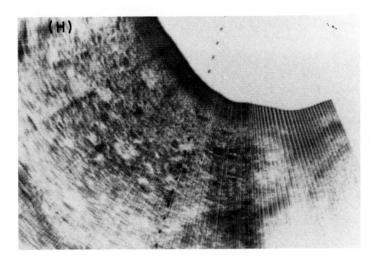

**Fig. 5-37.** Longitudinal scan. Diffuse pattern of "lucent" metastasis.

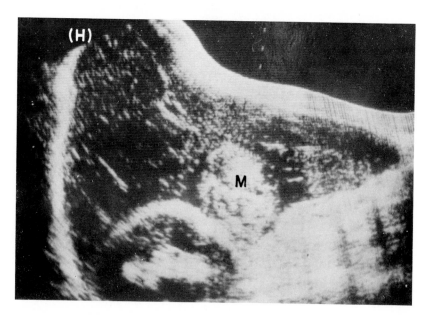

**Fig. 5-38.** Longitudinal scans. Note echogenic lesion (M).

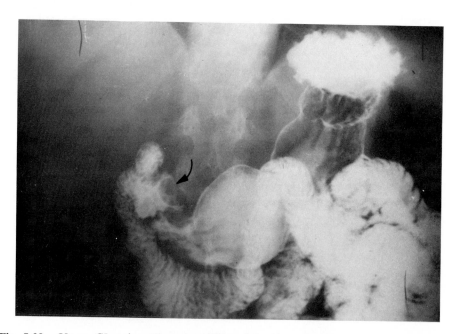

**Fig. 5-39.** Upper GI series. There is a filling defect identified within the duodenal bulb (arrows).

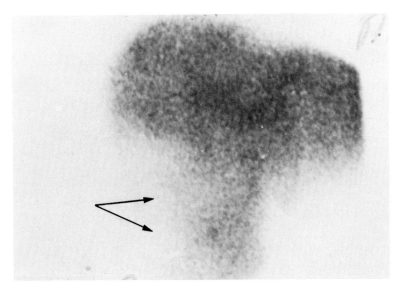

**Fig. 5-40.** Sulfur colloid liver scan—anterior view. Note focal defect (arrow).

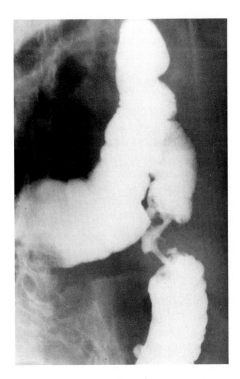

**Fig. 5-41.** Barium enema showing "apple-core" lesion.

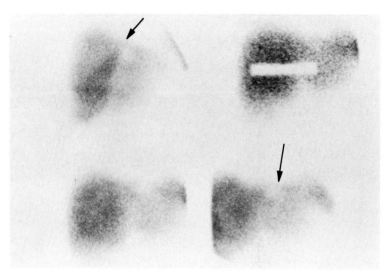

**Fig. 5-42.**    Sulfur colloid liver scan. Note focal defect at junction of the right and left lobes of the liver (arrow).

lesion is very well defined, and there is increased through transmission. These findings are characteristic of a simple hepatic cyst.

A follow-up study performed approximately one year later revealed no change in the appearance of this lesion.

## SUMMARY

Liver sonography serves as a useful complementary study to the radionuclide sulfur colloid liver scan. Because of the echogenic nature of the normal liver parenchyma, fluid-filled lesions within the liver, such as abscesses, are clearly identified. Before making the diagnosis of abscess or cyst, one must be certain that the sonolucent structure does not represent a dilated gallbladder.

Fluid collections around the liver, such as subphrenic abscesses, can be effectively evaluated by means of sonography. Fluid in such cases is located between the right hemidiaphragm and liver, as compared to right pleural effusions in which the fluid is, obviously, above the right hemidiaphragm. Also, the length of excursion of the right hemidiaphragm may be evaluated by means of sonography.

Minimal ascites can be identified as collections of fluid around the liver, around the root of the mesentery, and adjacent to the urinary bladder. The cirrhotic liver presents sonographically as increased echogenicity within the liver parenchyma. The findings of ascites, increased echogenicity of the liver parenchyma, and a normal biliary tree in a jaundiced patient is characteristic of hepatocellular, rather than obstructive, disease.

Metastatic disease to the liver has a variety of presentations. The so-called bulls-eye lesion presents as slightly more echogenic than the normal liver paren-

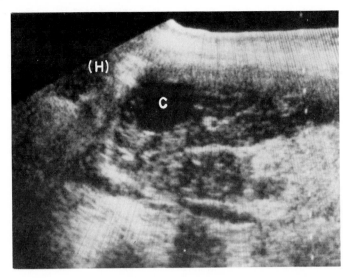

**Fig. 5-43.** Longitudinal scan showing hepatic cyst (C).

chyma and is surrounded by a sonolucent rim. Lesions more echogenic than the liver parenchyma are frequently seen in metastatic disease from the colon. The dense lesion presented on page 118 is a metastatic carcinoid. Another common variety of metastasis is the relatively sonolucent lesion. Multiple small sonolucent lesions result in the so-called diffuse pattern of metastasis.

## REFERENCES

1. Bryan PJ, Dinn WM: Isodense masses on CT: Differentiation by gray scale ultrasonography. Am J Roentgenol 129:989–922, 1977
2. Stephens DH, Sheedy PF, Hattery RR, et al: Computed tomography of the liver. Am J Roentgenol 128:579–590, 1977
3. Taylor, KJW, Atlas of gray scale ultrasonography. New York, Churchill Livingstone, 1978, p. 23.
4. Ibid, p. 16–18
5. Gerzof SG, Robbins AH, Birkett DH: Computed tomography in the diagnosis and management of abdominal abscesses. Gastrointest Radiol (In press)
6. Taylor, op. cit., pp 72–73
7. Garrett WJ, Kossoff G, Uren RF, et al: Gray scale ultrasonic investigation of focal defects on 99mTc sulfur colloid liver scanning. Radiology 119:425–428, 1976
8. Green B, Bree RL, Goldstein HM, et al: Gray scale ultrasound evaluation of hepatic neoplasm: Patterns and correlations. Radiology 124:203–208, 1977
9. McArdle CR: Ultrasonic diagnosis of liver metastases. J Clin Ultrasound 4:265–268, 1976
10. Scheible W, Gosink BB, Leopold GR: Gray scale echographic patterns of hepatic metastatic disease. Am J Roentgenol 129:983–987, 1977
11. Taylor KJW, Sullivan D, Rosenfield AT, et al: Gray scale ultrasound and isotope scanning: Complementary techniques for imaging the liver. Am J Roentgenol 128:227–281, 1977

# 6
# Renal Sonography

It should be stated at the outset that the intravenous pyelogram (IVP) remains the *sine qua non* of any renal workup. Some clinicians, overly enthusiastic about ultrasound, order renal sonography as the initial imaging study. There is great danger in attempting to interpret a renal sonogram without the benefit of an IVP. There are subtle changes that one may see on an IVP that cannot be visualized on a renal sonogram no matter how sophisticated the equipment may be. On the other hand, renal sonography does have a place in the overall workup of renal problems. As we shall see, there are situations in which renal ultrasound performs a very vital role.

## INDICATIONS

1. *Characterization of renal masses seen on IVP or KUB.* The distinction between solid and cystic renal masses has always been a dilemma. The early pioneering work of Goldberg and others with bistable and A-mode equipment helped to solve this problem. With the more sophisticated equipment available today, we can be even more accurate in our tissue characterization of renal masses.

2. *Ultrasonic guidance of renal cyst puncture.* Performed with or without the biopsy transducer, ultrasound provides an excellent means of directing the cyst puncture needle.

3. *Evaluation of the nonfunctioning kidney on IVP.* This has been found to be a surprisingly useful study. An attempt is made to ultrasound the patient between the 10-minute and delayed IVP films. Frequently, the pathology is identified so that delayed IVP films are unnecessary.

4. *Evaluation of the right upper quadrant masses.* In some patients, the lower pole of the right kidney lies in a very anterior position and can be palpated. Ultrasound provides a quick and effective means of detecting this particular anatomic variation (Fig. 6-1).

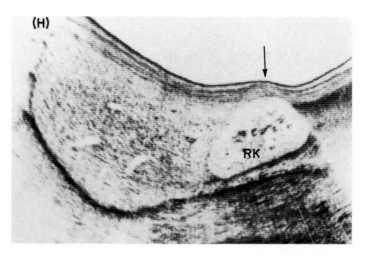

**Fig. 6-1.** Supine longitudinal scan. The lower pole of the right kidney could be palpated in this patient (arrow).

Even without these indications, familiarity of the sonographic anatomy and pathology of the kidneys is important. As described in Chapter 1, visualization of portions of the kidneys is a routine part of the basic abdominal examination. Parts of the left kidney are seen in the transverse sections, while the right kidney is seen in both transverse and longitudinal planes. The right kidney is especially scrutinized during a routine gallbladder sonogram. In many patients, the gallbladder lies in the same sagittal plane as the right kidney and may even be adjacent to it (Fig. 6-2). Frequently, stones in the gallbladder cast their shadows through the right kidney (Fig. 6-3). A whole gamut of renal pathology has been discovered, including renal cysts, tumors, and hydronephrosis, during routine gallbladder sonography.

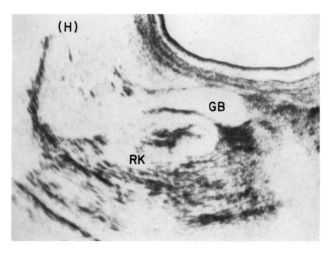

**Fig. 6-2.** Longitudinal scan. Note relationship of gallbladder to right kidney.

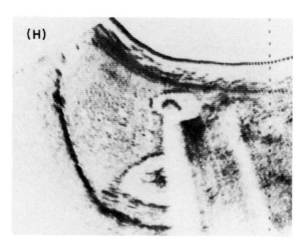

**Fig. 6-3.** Longitudinal scan. Gallstone causing shadowing through the right kidney (RK).

## TECHNIQUE

Because of the position of the kidneys, the basic abdominal sonogram described in Chapter 1 cannot be used. Instead, the patient is examined in the prone position. Compound transverse scans are obtained at 1 cm intervals from the top of the left kidney to the bottom of the right. A typical transverse scan is shown below. (Fig. 6-4).

The technician marks out the longitudinal axis of both kidneys on the patient's skin, and then proceeds with longitudinal cuts. Optimal longitudinal scanning is prevented by the presence of ribs between the transducer and the kidneys. This problem can, in part, be eliminated by adding sagittal sector scans of portions

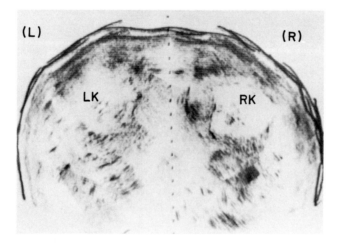

**Fig. 6-4.** Prone transverse scan.

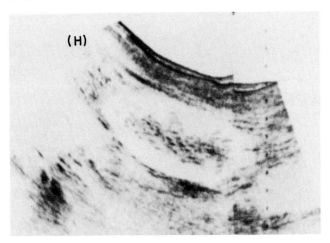

**Fig. 6-5.** Prone longitudinal scan.

of the kidneys together, which are obtained through different rib interspaces. The end result is a longitudinal view of the complete kidney (Fig. 6-5).

One-half centimeter longitudinal sections are then taken in both directions from the central longitudinal axis and until the kidney is no longer seen. Additional longitudinal views of the right kidney are obtained in the supine or semidecubitus position using the liver as a window (Fig. 6-6). It is in this projection that the renal anatomy may be best appreciated. The central clump of echoes represents the collecting system. The relatively sonolucent portion around the collecting system represents the renal parenchyma, cortex, and medulla.

The medulla is relatively sonolucent and, in patients with diminished peripelvic fat, appears not unlike a clump of small cysts encircling the collecting system

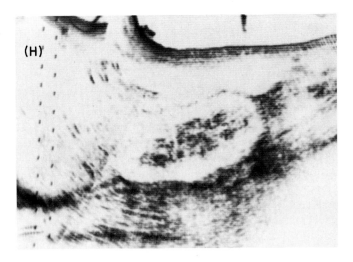

**Fig. 6-6.** Semidecubitus longitudinal scan of the right kidney.

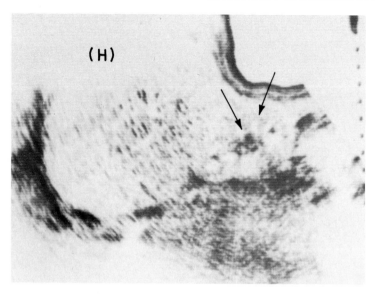

**Fig. 6-7.** Longitudinal scan of the right kidney. Note small sonolucent areas (arrows) adjacent to the collecting system.

(Fig. 6-7, arrows). The cortex is somewhat more echogenic than the medulla, but less so than the collecting system. For a more detailed description of intrarenal anatomy, the reader is referred to a paper by Cook, Rosenfield, and Taylor.[1]

Occasionally a discrete transverse separation of the central clump of echoes may be identified (Fig. 6-8). This represents a double collecting system.

Depending on the indications, one might desire supine transverse scans, such as those outlined in Chapter 1. Using the liver on the right and spleen on the left as windows, these scans can offer useful anatomic information. Finally, longitudinal decubiti scans may be useful when other methods fail. Again the liver on the right and spleen on the left are used as windows, and the transducer is angled up under the ribs.

## RENAL CYSTS

Any radiologist who routinely interprets IVPs will attest to the frequency with which simple renal cysts are discovered. It was not until the advent of ultrasound, however, that the radiologist could fully appreciate just how common these cysts are. Often they are discovered during unrelated examinations; the gallbladder sonogram is a prime example.

The classical renal cyst (Fig. 6-9) is totally sonolucent, attenuates nearly no sound, and presents sharp boundaries with the normal portions of the kidney

If the contents of a renal cyst present anything but a totally sonolucent appearance, one should become suspicious of the possibilities of hemorrhage,

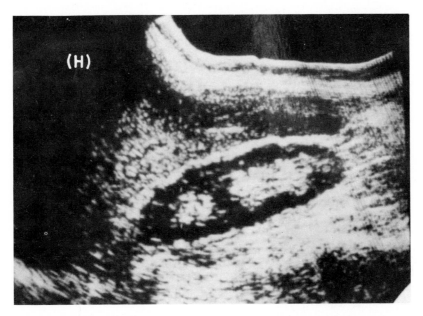

**Fig. 6-8.** Longitudinal scan of the right kidney. Duplicated collecting system.

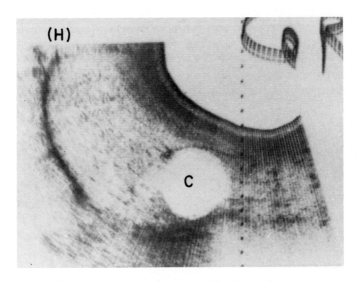

**Fig. 6-9.** Longitudinal scan. Simple renal cyst.

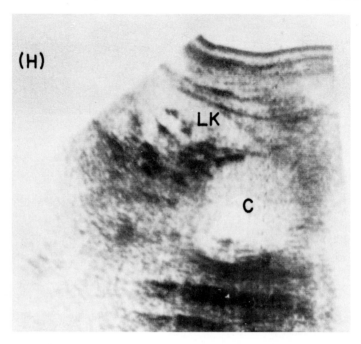

**Fig. 6-10.** Prone longitudinal scan of the left kidney. Cyst (C) "fills in" because of improper technique.

infection, or tumor. Technique, therefore, is quite important. A prone longitudinal scan of a simple renal cyst that becomes complicated because of maladjustment of the gain and TGC curves is shown (Fig. 6-10). Although simple renal cysts do not contain urine, their composition is very much like urine and should possess the same sonographic characteristics. It is, therefore, useful to compare the echogenicity of the renal cyst to the contents of the urinary bladder when there is doubt.

A calcified simple renal cyst (Fig. 6-11A, 6-11B) is very similar to the noncalcified variety, except that the walls appear to be somewhat thicker (arrows).

The presence of debris within a cyst raises the specter of neoplasm. One cannot be 100 percent certain that a cyst, even with all the features of a classical simple cyst, does not represent a renal neoplasm. The presence of such lesions as large cavitating hypernephromas and small tumor implants on the walls of cysts with reported incidences of between 1 and 7 percent[2], should make us reluctant to rule out the possibility of tumor. Since renal carcinomas are one of the most amenable tumors to treatment, it would be tragic, indeed, if one were missed in its early stages.

So the problem is not so much how to find renal cysts (plenty are found), but what to do with them once they are discovered. As physicians interpreting ultrasound images and IVPs, we find ourselves in the middle of a long-standing contro-

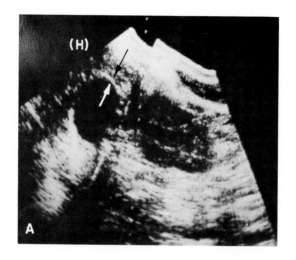

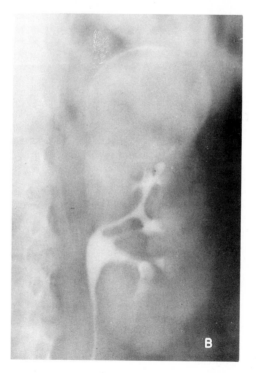

**Fig. 6-11.** (A) Prone longitudinal scan. Note thickened walls of cyst (arrows). (B) IVP.

versy. The techniques of ultrasonically or fluoroscopically guided percutaneous cyst puncture have helped to resolve this problem to some extent. In a review of 5674 cases of percutaneous cyst punctures, Lang reported a 1.4 percent mean incidence of major complications.[3] The incidence of major complications in institutions with extensive experience was approximately 0.75 percent. There is, therefore, a small but definite risk in achieving the high level of diagnostic accuracy that is afforded by this procedure. Certainly one should consider such factors as the size and position of the cyst, the age and overall condition of the patient, and so on. The advisability, therefore, of performing percutaneous cyst puncture should be evaluated on a case-by case basis.

### Case

DM is a 52-year-old female admitted for workup of hypertension. Below are prone longitudinal scans of both kidneys (Fig. 6-12, 6-13).

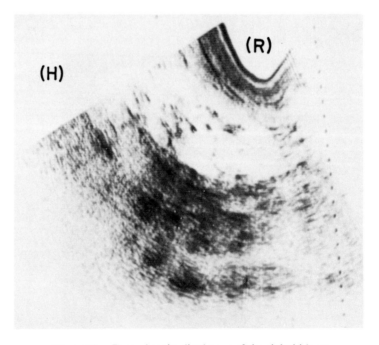

**Fig. 6-12.** Prone longitudinal scan of the right kidney.

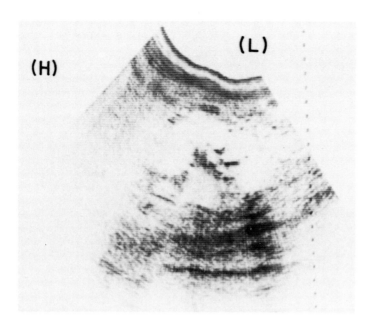

**Fig. 6-13.** Prone longitudinal scan of the left kidney.

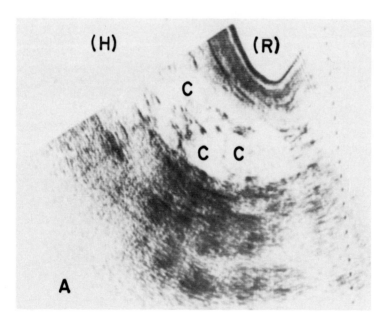

**Fig. 6-14 A.** Prone longitudinal scan of the right kidney.

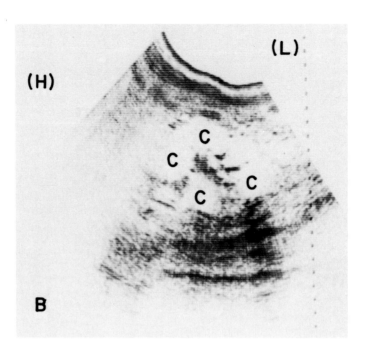

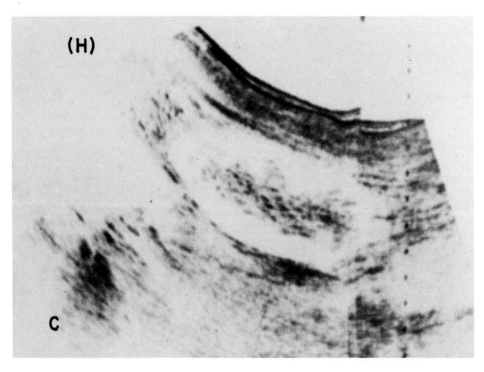

**Fig. 6-14 (B and C).** (B) Prone longitudinal scan of the left kidney. (C) Prone longitudinal scan of a normal kidney.

DISCUSSION

The prone longitudinal scans of both kidneys (Fig. 6-14A, 6-14B) reveal the presence of multiple, small intrarenal cysts (C). The cysts appear to involve the entire kidney, including the cortex and medulla, and also seem to impinge upon the collecting system echoes. Compare this scan to the normal kidney in Fig. 6-14C.

FOLLOW UP

An IVP (Fig. 6-15) reveals x-ray changes characteristic of polycystic kidney disease.

COMMENTS

1.  Ultrasound provides a convenient means of following patients with polycystic kidney disease, particularly in cases where renal function is inadequate for intravenous urography.

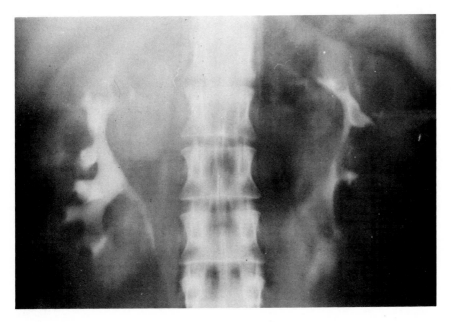

**Fig. 6-15.**   IVP.

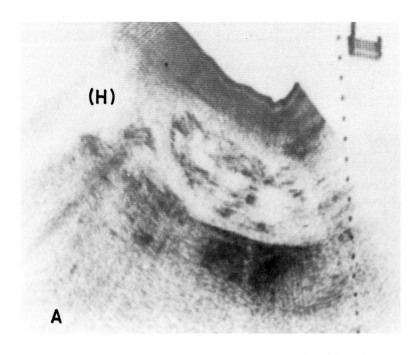

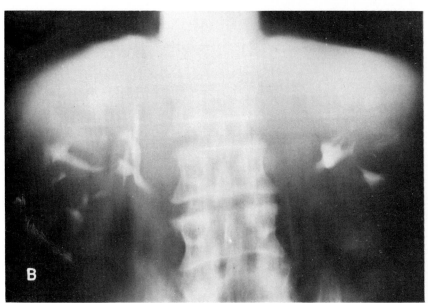

**Fig. 6-16.** (A) Prone longitudinal scan of the left kidney. (B) IVP.

2. Page 134 is a prone longitudinal scan of the left kidney (Fig. 6-16A) in another patient. An IVP film is also reproduced (Fig. 6-16B). How would you interpret the sonogram in the light of the IVP?

This case falls into the second category of renal pelvic lipomatosis described by Yeh, Mitty, and Wolf.[4] As compared to hydronephrosis and multiple peripelvic cysts, the small sonolucent areas seen in this case (Fig. 6-17C) represent small areas of fat deposition rather than fluid-filled spaces. As a result, these areas of fat are weakly echogenic and tend to attenuate sound to some extent. Nevertheless, the distinction between this entity and early hydronephrosis is difficult to achieve sonographically.

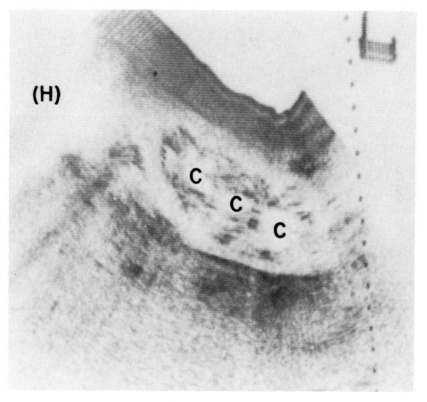

**Fig. 6-17.** Prone longitudinal scan of the left kidney. Note multiple cyst-like (C) lesions within the collecting system.

### Cases A–D

JK is a 66-year-old male referred to our department for gallbladder sonography. His gallbladder was normal. Longitudinal semidecubitus and prone longitudinal scans are shown below (Fig. 6-18, 6-19, 6-20). What is your provisional diagnosis and how would you proceed with further workup?

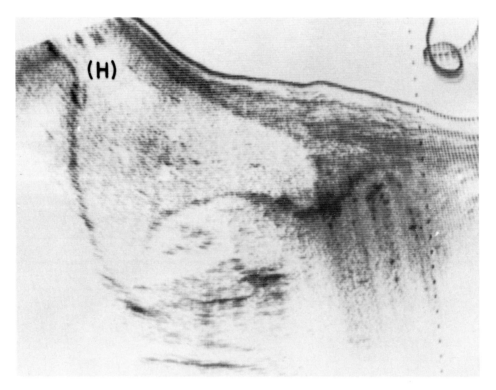

**Fig. 6-18.**  Semidecubitus longitudinal scan.

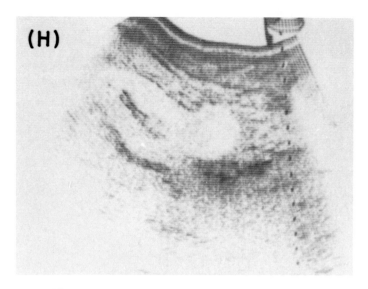

**Fig. 6-19.** Prone longitudinal scan of the right kidney.

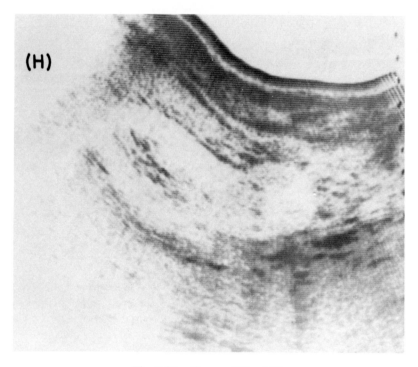

**Fig. 6-20.** Zoom of Fig. 6-19.

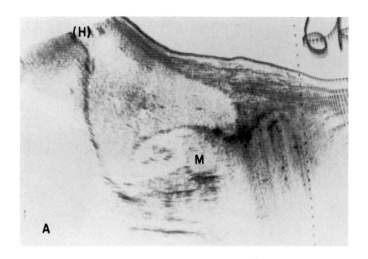

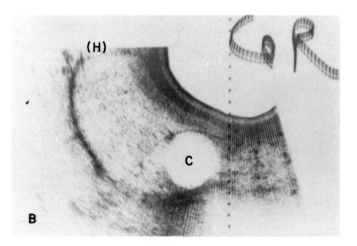

**Fig. 6-21.** (A) Semidecubitus longitudinal scan. Note mass (M) projecting off the lower pole of the right kidney. (B) Longitudinal scan. Simple renal cyst.

DISCUSSION

The longitudinal semidecubitus scan (Fig. 6-21A) clearly reveals a mass (M) projecting off the lower pole of the right kidney. There is greater echo activity within this mass than in the adjacent renal parenchyma. Compare this case to the simple renal cyst in Figure 6-21B. The solid lesion has irregular margins, while the boundaries of the cyst are very well defined. In addition, there is more transmission of sound through the cyst.

A longitudinal semidecubitus scan of another solid renal tumor in Case B is reproduced in Fig. 6-22 (M). In this case, the solid mass appears to be impinging upon the collecting system. Note the echogenicity of the mass as compared to the relatively sonolucent renal parenchyma.

Case C reveals a solid renal mass projecting off the lower pole of the left kidney (Fig. 6-23A, M). Since this particular mass extends far laterally and posteriorly, it can be best appreciated on the transverse scan (Fig. 6-23B, M). Again, compare the echogenicity of the mass to the normal renal parenchyma.

FOLLOW UP

Selective renal arteriograms in the above three patients are reproduced below (Fig. 6-24A, 6-24B, 6-24C). All the lesions are quite vascular. The pathological diagnosis in these cases was hypernephroma.

COMMENTS

1. There are occasions in which sonographic evaluation of the kidneys provides information that may only be suspected on intravenous urography. This has been found to be the case particularly when dealing with the upper pole of the right kidney. The close anatomic relation of the upper pole of this organ to the liver makes radiographic evaluation of the upper pole somewhat difficult. On the contrary, the upper pole of the right kidney can be easily evaluated sonographically because of the excellent acoustic window provided by the adja-

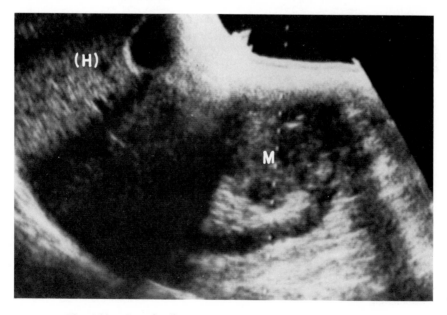

**Fig. 6-22.**   Longitudinal scan. Note echogenicity of mass (M).

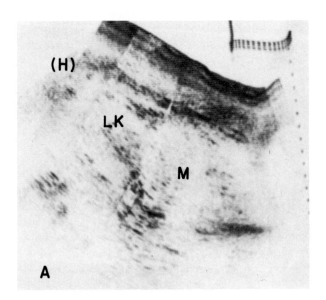

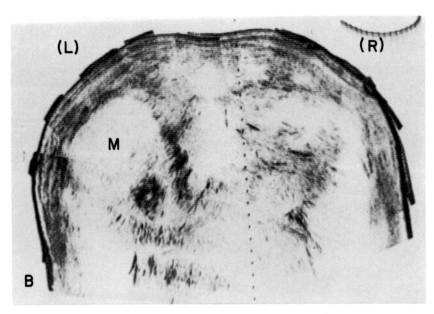

**Fig. 6-23.** (A) Prone longitudinal scan of the left kidney. A poorly defined mass (M) is projecting off the lower pole. (B) Prone transverse scan. The mass is better defined on the transverse section.

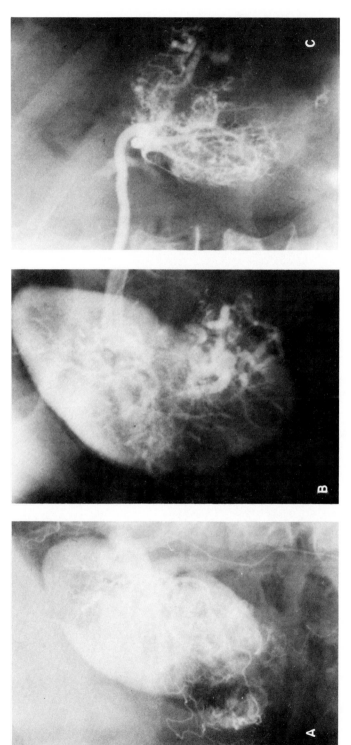

**Fig. 6-24.** Renal arteriograms in three cases reveal vascular masses. (A) Renal arteriogram of Case A. (B) Renal arteriogram of Case B. (C) Renal arteriogram of Case C.

141

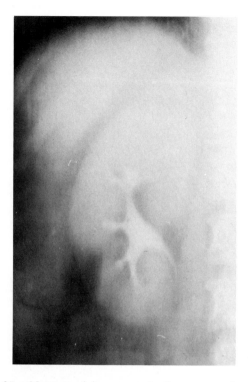

**Fig. 6-25.** Note suspicious mass in the upper pole of the right kidney.

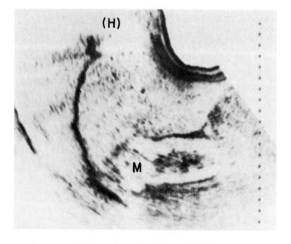

**Fig. 6-26.** Longitudinal scan. A well-defined mass (M) is seen involving the upper pole of the right kidney.

cent liver. In Case D (Fig.6-25, 6-26) a solid mass was suspected on the intravenous pyelogram. The mass is poorly defined and has no effect on the collecting system. The mass (M) is clearly defined on the longitudinal semidecubitus scan.

In Chapter 5, the role of liver sonography as a complementary procedure to the radionuclide liver scan was discussed. Certainly, a similar role for renal sonography as a complementary procedure to the intravenous pyelogram should be considered.

2.   In all these cases, the renal masses were moderately echogenic. Renal tumors, in general, have been reported to present with varying degrees of echogenicity. Some authors have correlated the echo-producing character of renal tumors with the vascularity of the lesion.[5] For example, avascular hypernephromas tend to be relatively sonolucent. Unlike simple cysts, however, these solid masses do attenuate sound and there is poor through transmission.

### Cases A and B

BL is a 65-year-old female who presented with ill-defined abdominal pain. A tomogram from her IVP is reproduced below (Fig. 6-27). Also shown below is a longitudinal semidecubitus scan of the right upper quadrant (Fig. 6-28). On the basis of the tomogram, what sort of pathology in the upper pole of the right kidney would you suspect? Does the sonogram confirm your suspicions?

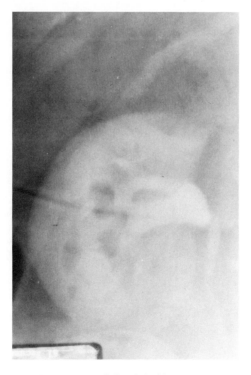

**Fig. 6-27.**   Tomogram of the right kidney from an IVP.

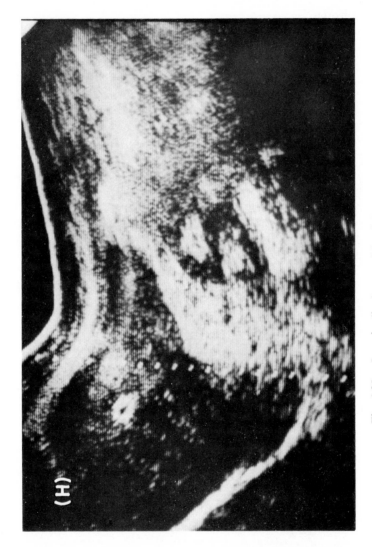

**Fig. 6-28.** Longitudinal scan of the right upper quadrant.

144

DISCUSSION

A cyst was suspected on the IVP. The mass appeared to be relatively radiolucent and there were well-defined claws. The mass on the longitudinal sonogram
(Fig. 6-29A, M) is somewhat difficult to evaluate anatomically ·It seems to be
between the upper pole of the right kidney and the liver. Compare Fig. 6-29A to
the normal right kidney in Fig. 6-29B. The type of tissue involved is more apparent. Certainly, one would not suspect a cyst. There is substantial echo activity
noted within the mass.

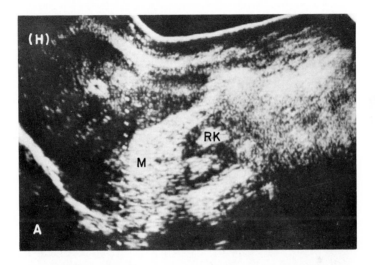

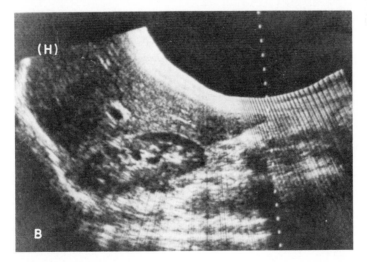

**Fig. 6-29.** (A) Longitudinal scan. There is an echogenic mass (M) between the right
kidney and the liver. (B) Longitudinal scan in normal patient.

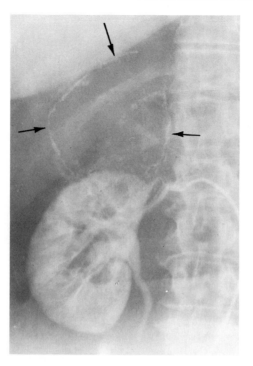

**Fig. 6-30.** Selective right renal arteriogram. Note irregular
artery coursing around periphery of the mass (arrows).

FOLLOW UP

A selective right renal arteriogram revealed a relatively avascular mass in the
upper pole (Fig. 6-30). There were, however, several abnormal vessels, one of
which was noted coursing around the periphery of the mass (arrows). At surgery,
an angiomyolipoma was encountered, The angiomatous component of the pathological specimen was minimal.

COMMENTS

1.  As mentioned in the beginning of this chapter, the IVP is the best single
    procedure for imaging the kidneys. One can be deceived, however, if one
    attempts to make a definive distinction between a solid mass and a cyst. The
    IVP in this case raised suspicions of a cyst, but other possibilities were
    quickly considered after the sonogram was viewed.
2.  The primary abnormality that was noted on the semidecubitus longitudinal
    scan in Case A (Fig. 6-31A) was increased echo activity between the upper
    pole of the right kidney and the liver. In normal patients, there is a fairly sharp
    interface between the upper pole of the right kidney and the liver (Fig. 6-31B).

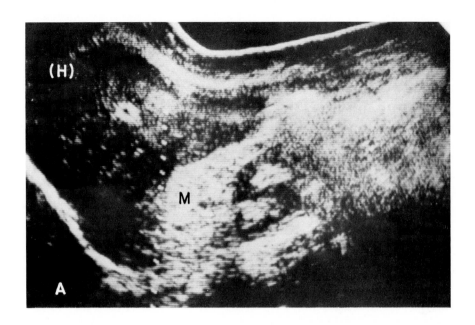

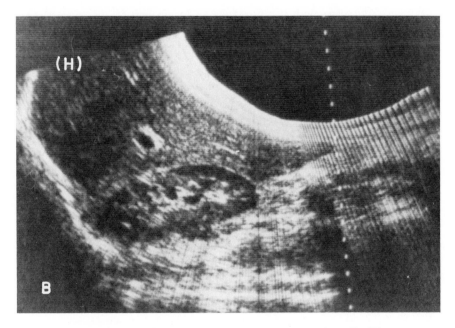

**Fig. 6-31.** (A) Longitudinal scan in patient BL (Case A). (B) Longitudinal scan in normal patient.

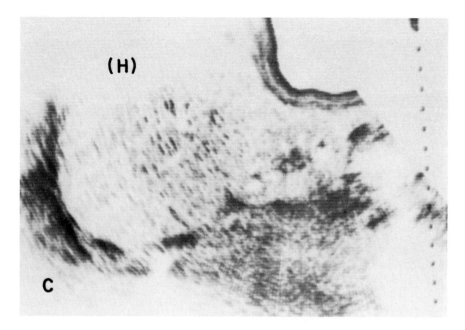

**Fig. 6-31C.** Longitudinal scan in Case B. The right kidney seems to blend with the liver parenchyma.

Taylor ascribes this acoustic interface to fascia and fat between the upper pole of the kidney and the lower edge of the liver. [6] The mass in Case A was composed primarily of fat, resulting in a wider echogenic interface.

In some patients, just the converse may be observed. The semidecubitus, longitudinal scan in Case B (Fig. 6-31C) reveals almost no interface between the kidney and the liver. This particular patient was emaciated and presumably had diminished fat content around the kidney. As a consequence, the renal parenchyma seems to blend into the liver parenchyma. The sonolucent pyramids of the kidneys also become more pronounced, presumably due to diminished fat content within the kidney itself.

### Case

MM is a 68-year-old female with a history of recent weight loss. An IVP with tomography revealed a mass projecting off the lower pole of the left kidney (Fig. 6-32, arrows). The mass appears relatively radiolucent. A radionuclide renal scan revealed absence of activity within the mass (Fig. 6-33). Prone transverse and longitudinal scans are shown below (Fig. 6-34, 6-35). Is the mass solid, cystic, or complex?

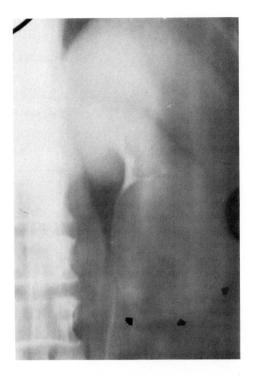

**Fig. 6-32.** Tomogram of the left kidney. Note mass projecting off the lower pole (arrows).

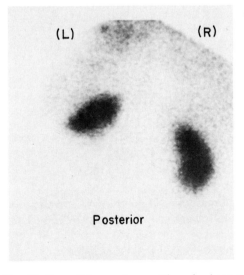

**Fig. 6-33.** Radionuclide renal scan. There is absence of activity in the lower pole of the left kidney.

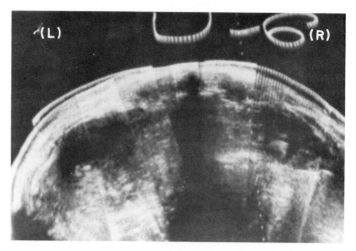

**Fig. 6-34.**    Prone transverse scan.

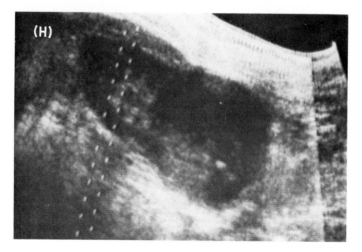

**Fig. 6-35.**    Prone longitudinal scan.

DISCUSSION

The prone longitudinal scan (Fig. 6-36A) reveals a predominantly sonolucent mass projecting off the lower pole of the left kidney. There is, however, echo activity in the anterior aspect of the mass (arrow), which would not go away. Many longitudinal scans revealed a solid component to the mass. Compare this mass to the cyst in Fig. 6-36B and the solid tumor in Fig. 6-36C. The mass is, therefore, complex. At this point, the following were considered as possibilities: Necrotic neoplasm, cyst with debris, and abscess.

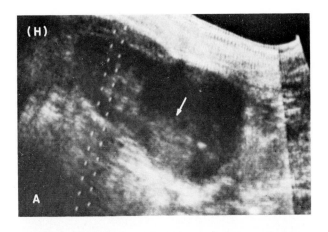

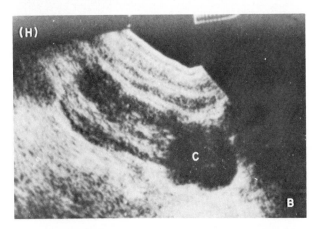

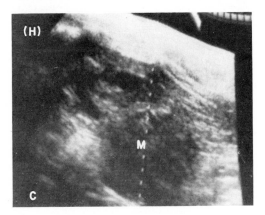

**Fig. 6-36.** (A) Prone longitudinal scan. There is echogenic material (arrow) within this predominantly sonolucent mass. (B) Prone longitudinal scan. Left lower pole renal cyst. (C) Prone longitudinal scan. Right lower pole hypernephroma.

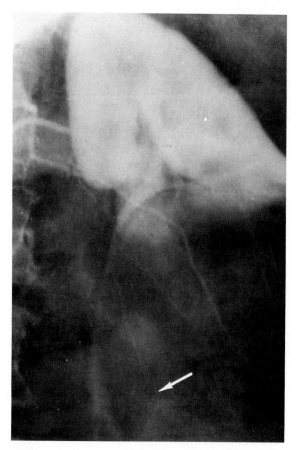

**Fig. 6-37.** Selective left renal arteriogram. The mass is avascular with the exception of a small collection of abnormal vessels (arrow).

FOLLOW UP

It was decided to proceed first with the renal arteriogram because neoplasm was high on the list of possibilities. (The patient had presented with significant weight loss.) A selective left renal arteriogram revealed an avascular mass in the lower pole (Fig. 6-37). There was, however, a small-caliber artery supplying a tiny collection of abnormal vessels within the mass (arrow).

Suspicion of a necrotic tumor persisted and a cyst puncture was performed. The patient's clinical condition was such that surgery was to be avoided if at all possible. The cyst puncture revealed an irregular "frondy" appearance to the cavity in the left lower pole (Fig. 6-38). The aspirate was bloody and positive for malignant cells. At surgery, a necrotic hypernephroma of the left kidney was encountered.

COMMENT

Evaluation of renal masses is one of the more common exams performed in our department. Generally, it is not a difficult matter to distinguish between solid

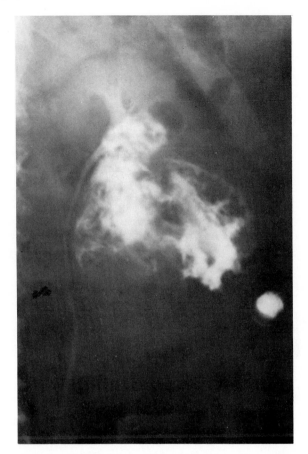

**Fig. 6-38.** Percutaneous "cyst" puncture. The confines of the mass present a "frondy" appearance.

and cystic masses. Complex masses, such as demonstrated in this case, require more care. Often, extraneous echoes, such as reverberations, present themselves in renal cysts. When they persist in several different scanning planes and after many scans, one should become suspicious of a solid component.

### Case

TP is a 55-year-old female admitted for workup of abdominal pain. A routine IVP revealed no evidence of function on the left (Fig. 6-39). There was no evidence of a pelvic kidney. The patient was sent for renal sonography while awaiting a delayed IVP film. Representative prone transverse and longitudinal scans are shown below (Fig. 6-40, 6-41, 6-42). Among the possibilities to be considered at this point would be nonfunction due to hydronephrosis, renal artery obstruction, multicystic dysplasia, or agenesis. Study the scans and try to find evidence for any of these conditions.

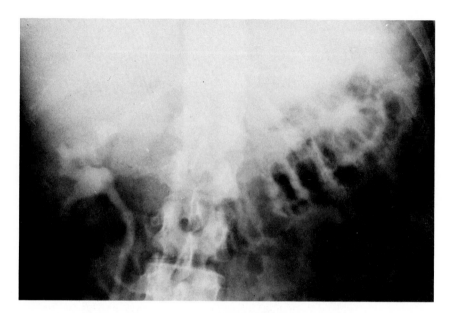

**Fig. 6-39.** IVP.

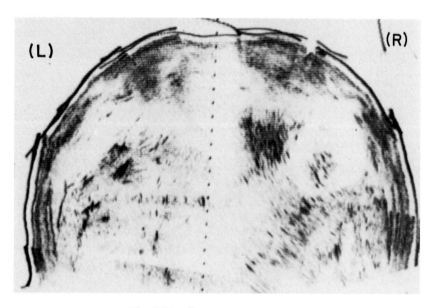

**Fig. 6-40.** Prone transverse scan.

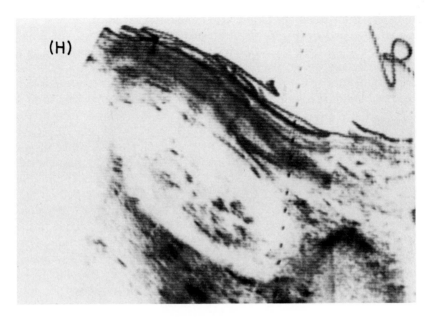

**Fig. 6-41.** Prone longitudinal scan on the right.

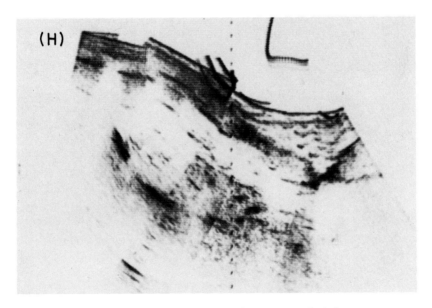

**Fig. 6-42.** Prone longitudinal scan on the left.

## DISCUSSION

The prone transverse scan reveals a normal renal outline on the right with a normal group of pelvocalyceal echoes (Fig. 6-43). On the left side there is no definite evidence of renal structure. The longitudinal scan of the left flank presents a confusing picture (Fig. 6-44). If you can envision a kidney, you are overusing your imagination. There is no kidney here. Instead, we are imaging structures other than the kidney which now fill the left renal fossa.

The longitudinal scans of the right kidney (Fig.6-41) reveal a normal sonographic appearance. This kidney, however, appears to be somewhat plump.

## FOLLOW UP

In this particular case, there is a radiographic clue to the cause of nonfunction. Teele et al. have described a sign of left renal agenesis.[7] In the absence of the left kidney, the splenic flexure of the colon "falls" into the the left renal fossa. If gas is present within the splenic flexure, this sign can be identified on the KUB (Fig. 6-45). The anatomic splenic flexure has fallen from its usual position under the left hemidiaphragm into the left renal fossa (arrow). This change in the position of the splenic flexure presents a confusing sonographic picture. Teele and associates described a "comma-shaped" appearance of the colonic mass in the left renal fossa (Fig. 6-44). Another clue is the "plump" sonographic appearance of the right kidney (Fig.6-41), presumably due to compensatory hypertrophy.

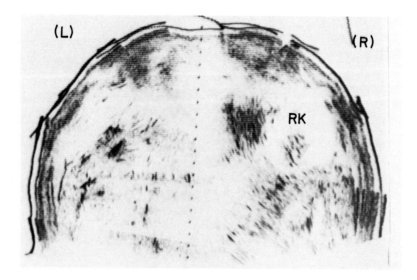

**Fig. 6-43.**   Prone transverse scan. Note normal right kidney.

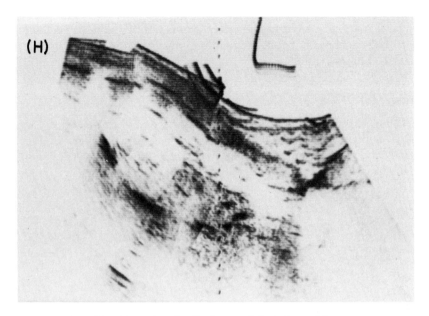

**Fig. 6-44.** Prone longitudinal scan of the left renal fossa.

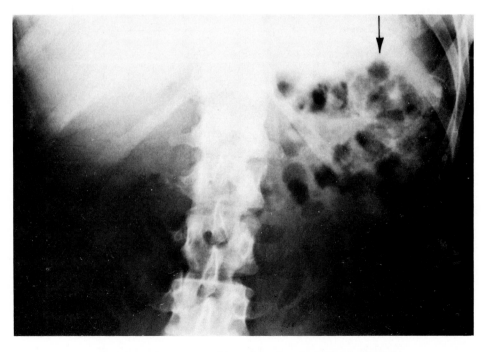

**Fig. 6-45.** KUB. Note position of gas in splenic flexure (arrow).

COMMENT

As mentioned in the introduction of this chapter, ultrasound provides a sur-prisingly effective means of studying the nonfunctioning kidney. Such causes as agenesis, hydronephrosis, neoplasm, and multicystic dysplasia may be identified by means of the renal sonogram.

### Case

HH is a 31-year-old female referred with right upper quadrant pain for a gallbladder sonogram. Her gallbladder was normal. Longitudinal semidecubitus and prone scans and a supine transverse scan are shown below (Fig. 6-46, 6-47, 6-48). Did the patient need an oral cholecystogram or an IVP?

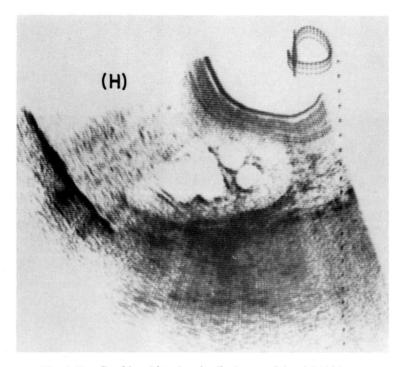

**Fig. 6-46.** Semidecubitus longitudinal scan of the right kidney.

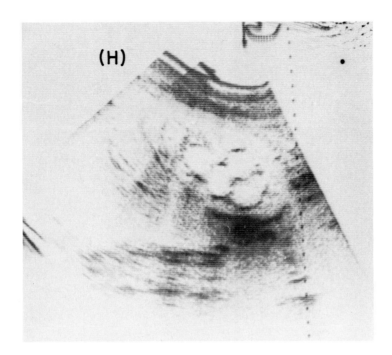

**Fig. 6-47.** Prone longitudinal scan of the right kidney.

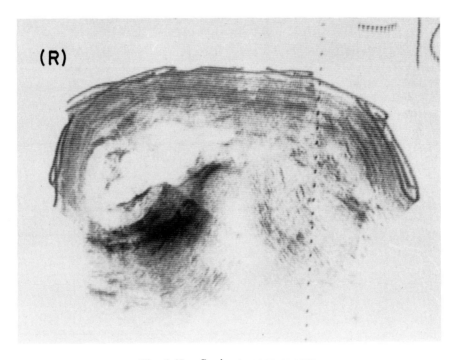

**Fig. 6-48.** Supine transverse scan.

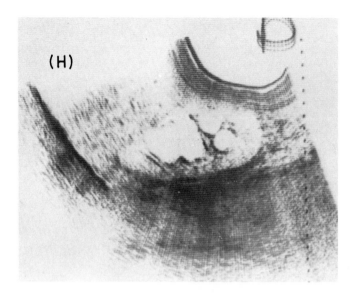

**Fig. 6-49.**   Semidecubitus longitudinal scan.

DISCUSSION

HH needed an IVP. The longitudinal scan (Fig. 6-49) reveals distortion of the collecting system echoes by multiple cystic lesions. The transverse scan (Fig. 6-50) reveals a dilated collecting system with a dilated renal pelvis. (P).

FOLLOW UP

An IVP revealed a right hydronephrosis secondary to a stone in the right distal ureter (Fig. 6-51).

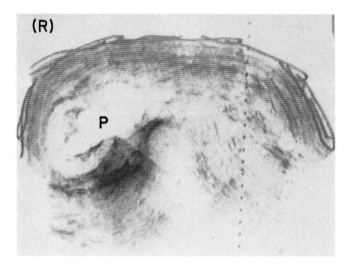

**Fig. 6-50.**   Supine transverse scan. The right renal pelvis (P) is dilated.

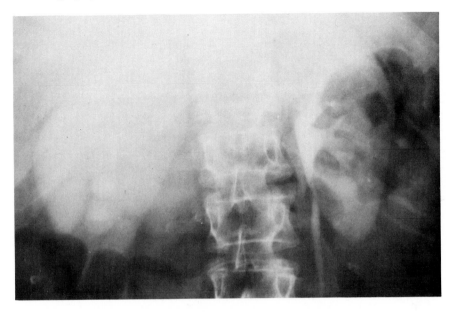

**Fig. 6-51.** IVP.

COMMENTS

1. In cases of early hydronephrosis, the calyceal structure may appear normal sonographically (Fig.6-52A). As one moves more medially, the dilated pelvis may be appreciated (Fig. 6-52B). Finally, a sagittal section taken 0.5 cm more medially (Fig.6-52C) reveals the dilated ureter (U).

2. An attempt to find the stone by means of ultrasound after the IVP was unsuccessful (Fig. 6-53). The dilated ureter was visible, although the stone was not.

Is there any value in attempting to find stones in the urinary tract by ultrasound? The vast majority (approximately 80 percent) of stones in the urinary tract are calcified and can be identified on a KUB. A recent report by Pollack and associates suggests that ultrasound may be valuable in the detection of nonopaque calculi, such as uric acid stones.[8] Our experience has included two uric acid stones. One stone was associated with a sharply defined acoustic shadow(Fig. 6-54, small arrows).

The other stone was in a patient who presented with hydronephrosis secondary to a mass in the renal pelvis. Being enthusiastic about ultrasound, the clinician referred the patient to us hoping that we would find the stone, and thereby eliminating more serious possibilities. The patient's affected kidney was scanned many times and did not demonstrate an acoustic shadow. The patient went to surgery and a uric stone was removed from the renal pelvis. The clinician called us immediately to question the value of the whole field of ultrasound. We, he claimed, failed to find the stone. I can only conclude that the stone simply did not

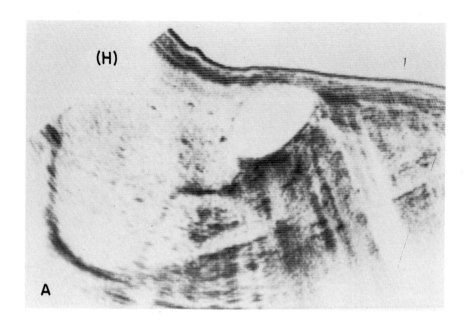

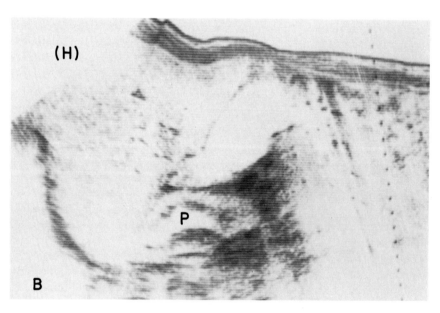

**Fig. 6-52.** (A) Longitudinal scan. Pelvocalyceal group of echoes appears normal in this section. (B) Longitudinal scan .05 cm more medial than 6-52A. The dilated renal pelvis (P) is now apparent.

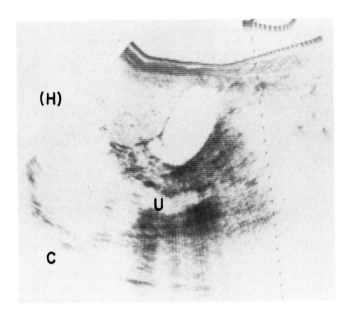

**Fig. 6-52C.** Longitudinal scan .05 cm more medial than 6-52B. The dilated ureter (U) can now be seen.

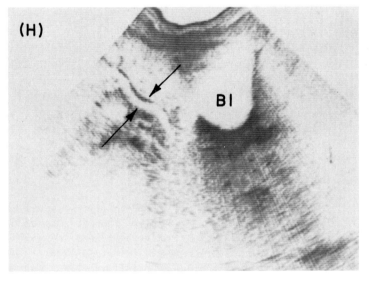

**Fig. 6-53.** Supine longitudinal scan. The dilated ureter (arrows) is seen approaching the urinary bladder (Bl).

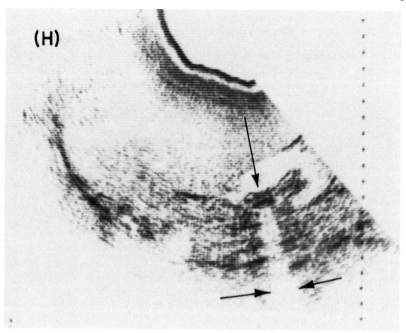

**Fig. 6-54.** Longitudinal scan. Note echogenic density within the right renal pelvis (large arrow) casting an acoustic shadow (small arrows).

shadow. To prove it, I went to great lengths to obtain the stone. I traveled to the patient's home, discussed his overall medical condition with him, and borrowed the stone that he kept proudly on his night table. I scanned the stone in vitro and could not get it to shadow. Finally, a friend at a large hospital in Connecticut borrowed the stone from me with the challenge that he could get it to shadow. That was over a year ago, and I have not heard from him. You may draw your own conclusions.

### Case

MM is a 69-year-old male admitted with right-sided abdominal pain. An IVP revealed non-function on the right. Tomograms, however, revealed multiple, large, ring-shaped calcifications in the area of the right kidney (Fig. 6-55, arrows). In retrospect, these calcifications were present on the plain film. Pages 165–166 are representative transverse and longitudinal prone sonograms (Figs. 6-56, 6-57, 6-58). Note that one of the transverse sonograms was taken just below the top of the left kidney, while the other was taken approximately 9 cm below the top of the left kidney. Can you deduce the etiology of nonfunction in this patient?

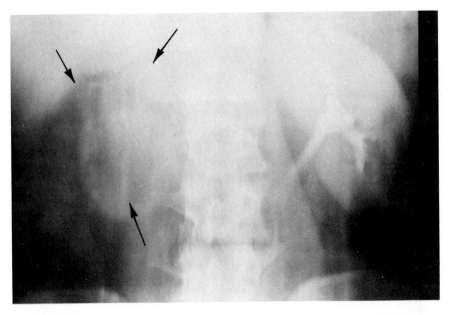

**Fig. 6-55.** IVP. Note faint ring-shaped calcifications (arrows) on the right.

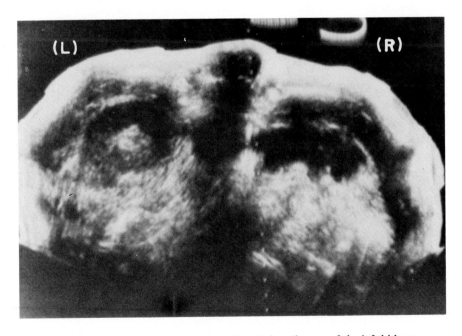

**Fig. 6-56.** Prone transverse scan at 5 cm below the top of the left kidney.

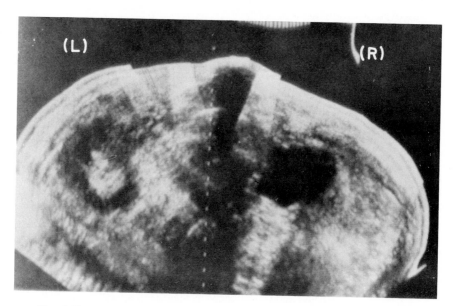

**Fig. 6-57.** Prone transverse scan at 9 cm below the top of the left kidney.

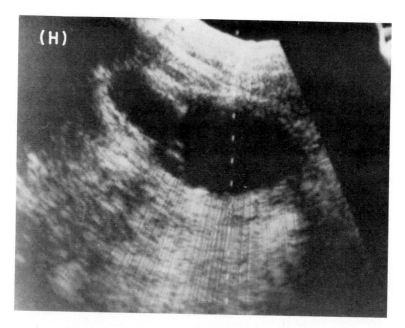

**Fig. 6-58.** Prone longitudinal scan of the right kidney.

166

DISCUSSION

No evidence could be found of a normal renal parenchyma on the right. The longitudinal sonogram (Fig. 6-59) revealed a large multiocular cyst.

The transverse sections, one at the top of the left kidney (Fig. 6-60A) and one at the bottom (Fig. 6-60B), also showed that the right renal fossa was filled with cysts. These large, multilocular cysts are somewhat difficult to evaluate with the sector scanner because of their size. This is another area where real time scanners are valuable. With a real time system, one can sweep through the entire cyst and better appreciate its appearance. With the sector scanner, one must mentally convert the longitudinal and transverse sections into a reasonable three dimensional picture.

FOLLOW UP

An atretic right ureter was found at cystoscopy. The postoperative diagnosis was multicystic dysplasia of the right kidney.

COMMENTS

Cases have been demonstrated in which multiple large cystic structures have represented severe chronic hydronephrosis. It is not surprising that these two conditions look alike in view of the prevalent theory that multicystic dysplasia is a hydronephrosis that occurs in utero. Indeed, some authors have made this in utero diagnosis by means of ultrasound. We have not done so yet, but we keep looking (Fig. 6-61). Incidentally, the lower portion of the genitourinary tract may also be nicely imaged in utero (Fig. 6-62).

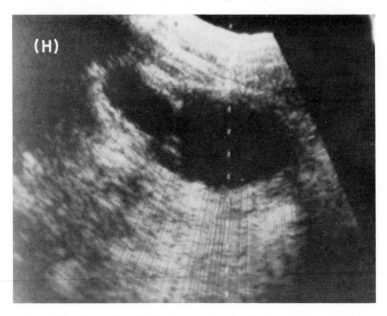

**Fig. 6-59.**   Prone longitudinal scan showing large sonolucent mass.

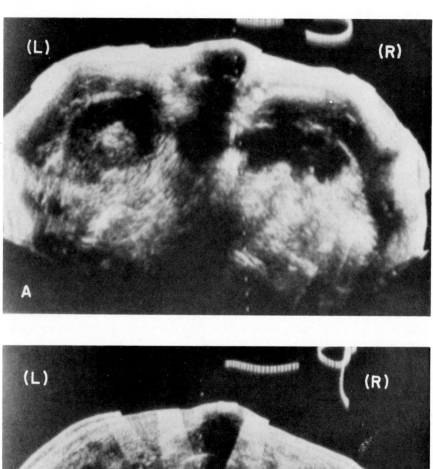

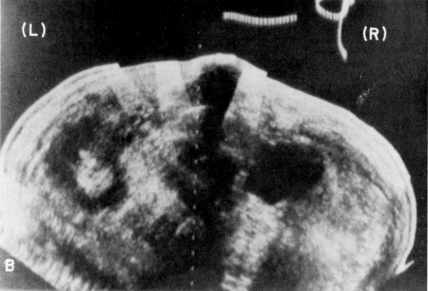

**Fig. 6-60.** (A) Prone transverse scan at xyphoid −5 cm. (B) Prone transverse scan at xyphoid −9 cm.

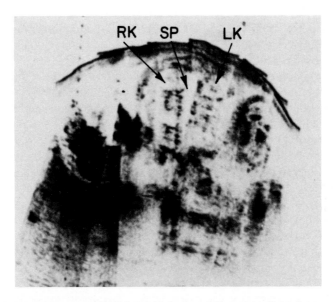

**Fig. 6-61.** Transverse scan of the fetal abdomen. The spine (Sp), right and left kidneys (RK, LK) are labeled.

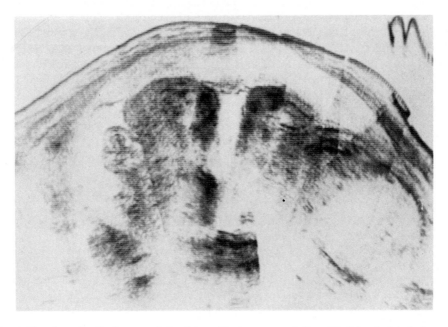

**Fig. 6-62.** Longitudinal scan of the fetus. Vertex presentation. Nothing is labeled—use your imagination.

## SUMMARY

Although renal sonography has a definite place in the overall workup of renal disease, it should not be considered a substitute, but a complementary procedure to the intravenous pyelogram. One of the prime uses of renal sonography is in the evaluation of masses identified on IVP or KUB. The classical renal cyst presents as a completely sonolucent lesion, which attenuates very little sound and which presents sharp boundaries with the normal portions of the kidney. Virtually 100 percent accuracy in making the diagnosis of simple renal cysts can be attained by ultrasonically or fluoroscopically guided cyst puncture.

Sonolucent renal masses with localized echo activity in the wall of the cyst raises the possibility of neoplasm and should be further studied by means of cyst puncture and/or arteriography. As compared to cysts, solid renal masses, such as hypernephromas, present as relatively echogenic lesions. When such lesions are encountered, further evaluation is indicated.

The pelvocalyceal portion of the normal kidney presents sonographically as a dense clump of echoes. The medulla, adjacent to the collecting system, often appears as multiple small sonolucent spaces. The cortex is somewhat more echogenic than the medula and is homogeneous. Renal pelvic lipomatosis presents as small, relatively sonolucent spaces within the pelvocalyceal clump of echoes. Polycystic kidney desease, on the other hand, frequently presents as multiple cysts involving both the collecting system and renal parenchyma.

Evaluation of the nonfunctioning kidney on IVP is another one of the major indications of renal sonography. Renal agenesis presents as absence of a recognizable kidney on the affected side. Hydronephrosis appears sonographically as separation of the pelvocalyceal group of echoes. If advanced, the normal kidney may be completely replaced by cystic structures. Ultrasound may also be effective in identifiying nonopaque renal calculi. Finally, the multicystic dysplastic kidney presents as multiple cysts which completely fill the renal fossa—a sonographic appearance not unlike advanced hydronephrosis.

## REFERENCES

1.  Cook JH, Rosenfield AT, Taylor KJ: Ultrasonic demonstration of intrarenal anatomy. Am J Roentgenol 129:831–834, 1977
2.  Emmet JL, Witten DM: Clinical urography. Vol 2 (ed 3), W. B. Saunders, Phila., 1971, p 32
3.  Lang EK: Renal cyst puncture and aspiration: A survey of complications. Am J Roentgenol 128:723–727, 1977
4.  Yeh H, Mitty HA, Wolf BS: Ultrasonography of renal sinus lipomatosis. Radiology 124:799–801, 1977
5.  Maklad NF, Chiang V, Doust BD: Ultrasonic characterization of solid renal lesion: Echographic, angiographic and pathologic correlation. Radiology 123:733–739, 1977
6.  Taylor KJW: Atlas of Gray Scale Ultrasonography. New York, Churchill Livingstone, 1978, p 30
7.  Teele R, Rosenfield AT, Freedman GS: The anatomic splenic flexure: An ultrasonic renal imposter. Am J Roentgenol 128:115–120, 1977
8.  Pollack HM, Aiger PH, Goldberg BB, et al: Ultrasonic detection of nonopaque renal calculi. Radiology 127:233–237, 1978

# 7
# Abdominal Aortic Aneurysms and Other Abdominal Conditions

Sonographic evaluation of the abdominal aorta has become a routine diagnostic procedure. The accuracy achieved by this examination is certainly an improvement over the more traditional methods, such as plain films of the abdomen. Contrast abdominal aortography also has its limitations because only the lumen of the aorta fills with contrast material. Ultrasonic evaluation, on the other hand, permits visualization of the lumen, as well as any clot that may be present around the lumen

## INDICATIONS

1. Evaluation of pulsatile abdominal masses.
2. Evaluation of masses suggested by other examinations, such as the KUB, IVP, etc.

## TECHNIQUE

Again the basic abdominal sonogram described in Chapter 1 serves as the backbone of the examination. The transverse scans (Fig. 7-1), however, are continued in a caudad direction until the aortic bifurcation is reached. Herein lies the problem. Unfortunately, bowel loops must be somewhere in the abdomen. In many patients, particularly those who are obese, they obscure much of the lower portion of the abdominal aorta. Because of tortousity of the abdominal aorta, it is usually helpful to map out the course of this vessel, while the transverse sections are taken. As a result, the sonographer is better able to understand the longitudinal course of the aorta. The longitudinal sweeps (Fig. 7-2) are taken at 0.5 cm intervals until the aorta is no longer visualized.

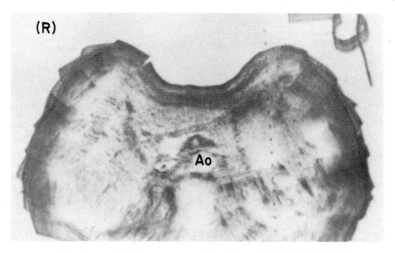

**Fig. 7-1.**  Transverse scan. The aorta (Ao) is labeled.

Aside from abdominal aortic aneurysms, other pathology in the lower abdomen may be evaluated by means of ultrasound. Masses, particularly in females, may arise in the pelvis and extend well up into the abdomen. Superficial abdominal masses, such as abscesses and hematomas, may also be evaluated. The technique used is, of course, dictated by the pathology that is present.

## ABDOMINAL AORTIC ANEURYSM

Most authors consider an abdominal aorta of 3 cm or more as aneurysm.[1] In our experience, aortic aneurysms without hematomas are the exception, rather than the rule. The clot, in general, is only a sonographic shade or two of gray

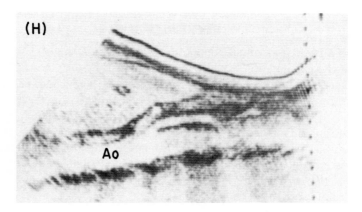

**Fig. 7-2.**  Longitudinal scan of the aorta (Ao).

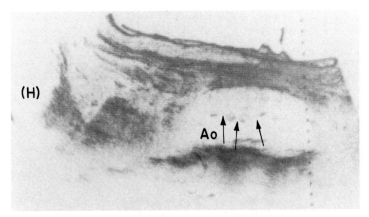

**Fig. 7-3.** Supine longitudinal scan. Note aneurysm and hematoma anteriorly (arrows).

different than the true lumen of the aorta. For this reason, it is essential to be sure that the equipment is properly adjusted and reverberation echoes eliminated. Fig. 7-3 and 7-4 below are examples of an aneurysm. Note that the clot in this case is anterior (arrows).

When the clot is in a more lateral position, it may be recognized only on the transverse scans. Below (Fig.7-5) is a transverse section from another patient. Note the size of the clot (C), as compared to the true lumen of the aorta (Ao). We have been able to appreciate these findings better with black background (Fig. 7-6).

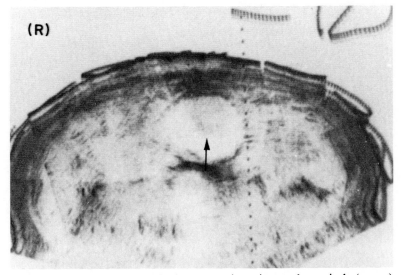

**Fig. 7-4.** Transverse scan. The hematoma is again noted anteriorly (arrow).

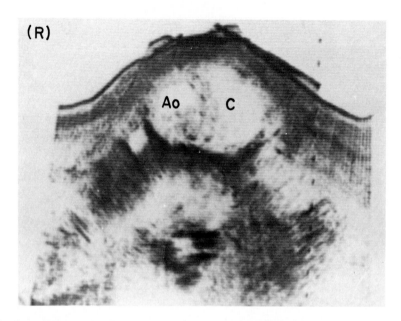

**Fig. 7-5.** Transverse scan. The clot (C) is large compared to the lumen of the aorta.

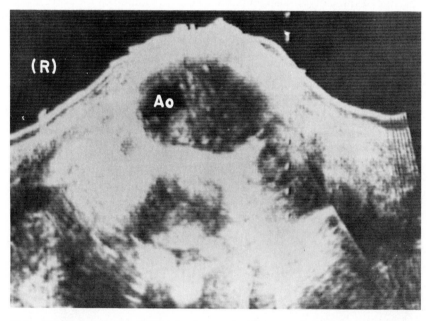

**Fig. 7-6.** Transverse scan—black background. The true lumen (Ao) can be better appreciated.

### Case

ST is a 53-year-old female who presented with weight loss and a palpable midabdominal mass. Below are typical transverse and longitudinal scans (Fig. 7-7, 7-8, 7-9). Is her abdominal aorta normal?

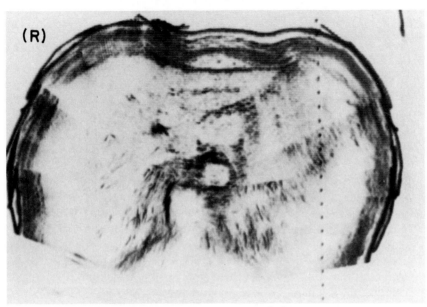

**Fig. 7-7.**   Transverse scan at xyphoid −1 cm.

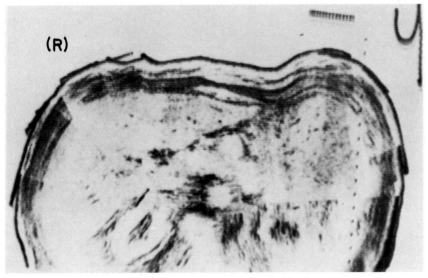

**Fig. 7-8.**   Transverse scan at xyphoid −2 cm.

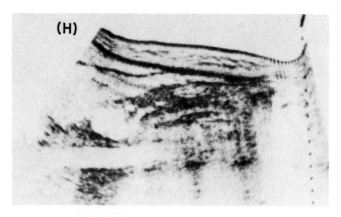

**Fig. 7-9.** Supine longitudinal scan over the aorta.

DISCUSSION

The transverse scan (Fig. 7-10) reveals a relatively sonolucent mass (M) anterior to the aorta (Ao). The mass is midline and extends toward the left. The aorta is normal and separate from this somewhat lobulated mass. The longitudinal scan (Fig. 7-11) confirms these findings. The mass (M) is anterior to the aorta (Ao).

FOLLOW UP

A gallium scan (Fig. 7-12) revealed uptake of the radionuclide in multiple areas including the left para-aortic region (arrows).

An IVP (Fig. 7-13) revealed lateral deviation of the left upper ureter (arrow). The patient had had a previous lymphangiogram, so the cause of the ureteral deviation is apparent

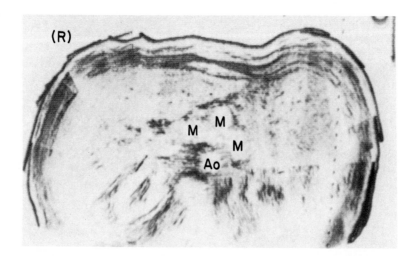

**Fig. 7-10.** Transverse scan at xyphoid −1 cm. There is a relatively sonolucent mass (M) anterior to the aorta (Ao).

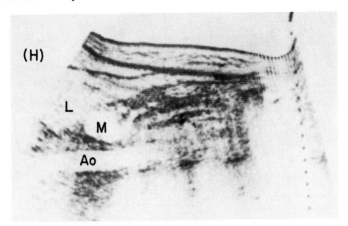

**Fig. 7-11.** Longitudinal scan. The mass (M) is just anterior to the aorta (Ao).

COMMENTS

1. Invaded lymph nodes around the aorta, particularly in lymphoma, may present sonographically as relatively lucent masses. The echo-producing character of the mass may, in fact, be very similar to the lumen of the aorta. Boundaries must, therefore, be identified before one is able to differentiate between an aneurysm and retroperitoneal mass, such as lymphoma.

2. Ultrasound provides a noninvasive means of studying the efficacy of treatment of lymphomas and other retroperitoneal neoplasms. For example, the patient FD presented with a large, hard abdominal mass. A KUB (Fig. 7-14) revealed a large soft tissue mass displacing loops of bowel (arrows).

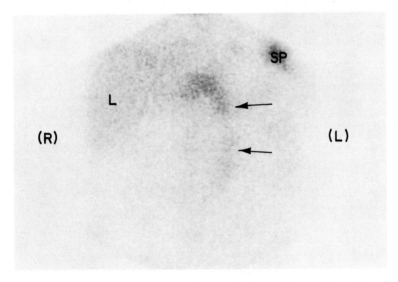

**Fig. 7-12.** Gallium scan—72 hours. Note uptake of radionuclide and liver (L), spleen (Sp), and para-aortic nodes (arrows).

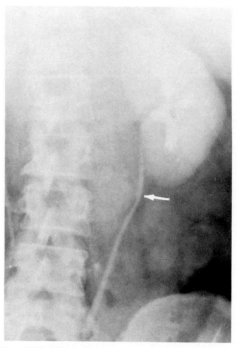

**Fig. 7-13.** IVP. There is lateral deviation of the left upper ureter (arrow).

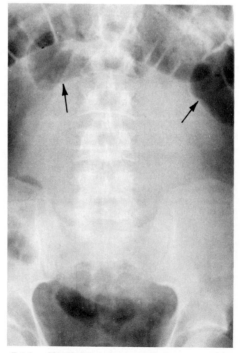

**Fig. 7-14.** KUB. Note large soft tissue mass (arrows).

178

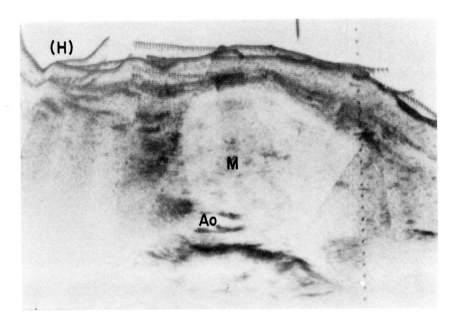

**Fig. 7-15.** Supine longitudinal scan. The solid mass (M) is anterior to the aorta (Ao).

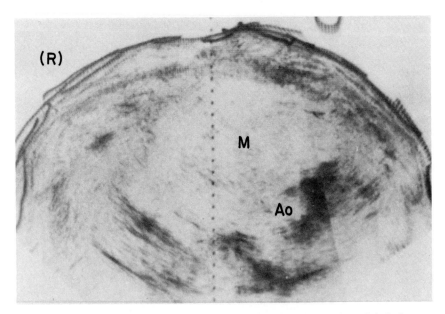

**Fig. 7-16.** Transverse scan. The mass (M) and aorta (Ao) are labeled.

179

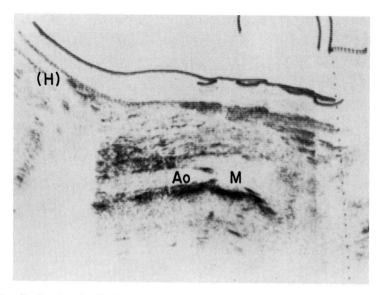

**Fig. 7-17.** Supine longitudinal scan. After treatment, the mass (M) has become much smaller. Compare to Fig. 7-15.

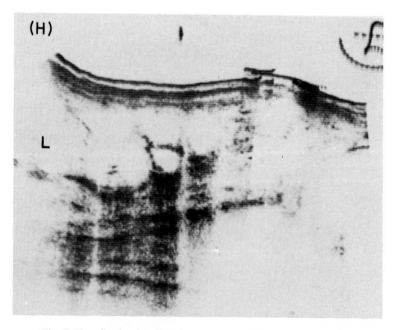

**Fig. 7-18.** Supine longitudinal scan. The liver (L) is labeled.

Representative longitudinal and transverse scans are shown on p. 179 (Fig. 7-15, 7-16). The mass (M) is solid and intimately related to the aorta. (Ao).

At surgery, a retroperitoneal sarcoma was encountered. The patient was treated and returned for a repeat sonogram approximately six months later. A longitudinal sonogram from the repeat study is shown below (Fig. 7-17). The mass (M) again appears to be intimately associated with the lower portion of the abdominal aorta and has become much smaller in size.

### Case

ZP is a 30-year-old female with fever and abdominal tenderness. Opposite are two representative longitudinal sonograms (Fig. 7-18, 7-19). The liver (L) bladder (B), and uterus (Ut) are labeled. A pertinent bit of history is being withheld.

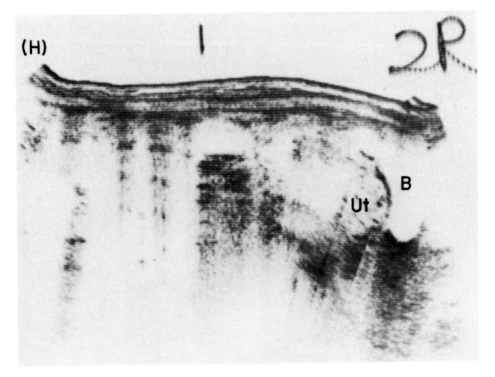

**Fig. 7-19.**    Supine longitudinal scan. The bladder (B) and uterus (Ut) are labeled.

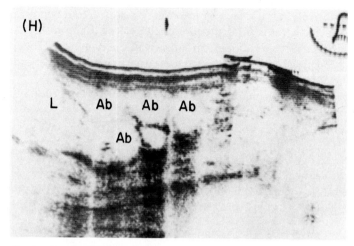

**Fig. 7-20.** Supine longitudinal scan. There are multiple superficial abscess cavities (Ab).

DISCUSSION

The longitudinal scan (Fig. 7-20) reveals multiple cystic lesions (Ab) within the anterior portion of the abdomen and adjacent to the uterus (Fig. 7-21). The transverse scans (not shown) confirm these findings. The history that was omitted was that the patient had had an appendectomy one week prior to the study.

FOLLOW UP

At surgery, multiple small abscesses were found.

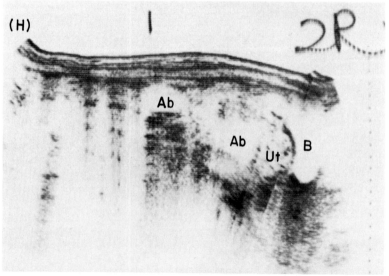

**Fig. 7-21.** Supine longitudinal scan. Note abscess cavities (Ab) anteriorly and cephalad to the uterus (Ut).

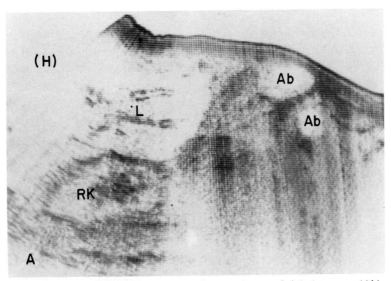

**Fig. 7-22A.** Longitudinal scan showing small superficial abscesses (Ab).

COMMENTS

Abdominal abscesses that occur postoperatively or are associated with diverticulitis may frequently be studied by means of ultrasound. The abscesses must, of course, be anterior to the gas within the bowel. This case is an example of an abscess that was associated with diverticulitis (Fig. 7-22A, Ab).

A follow-up study performed one week later (Fig. 7-22B) revealed some decrease in the size of the abscess (Ab).

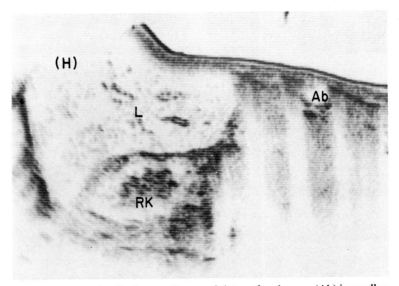

**Fig. 7-22B.** Longitudinal scan. One week later, the abscess (Ab) is smaller.

184

## Case

KG is a 47- year- old female with lower abdominal pain and a palpable lower abdominal mass. Below are longitudinal and transverse sonograms of her lower abdomen (Fig. 7-23, 7-24). Can you explain the patient's symptoms and physical findings on the basis of these scans?

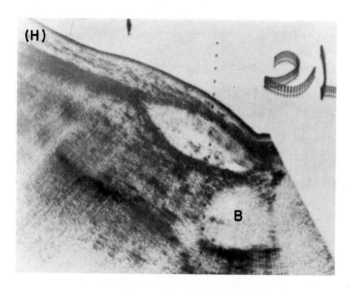

**Fig. 7-23.** Supine longitudinal scan. The bladder (B) is labeled.

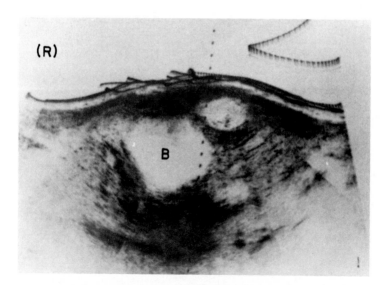

**Fig. 7-24.** Transverse scan. The bladder (B) is labeled.

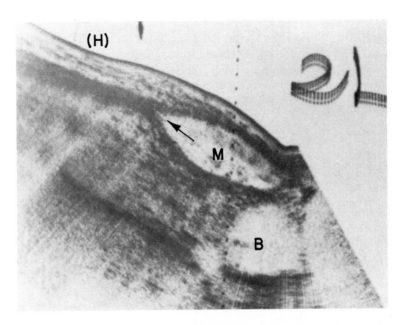

**Fig. 7-25.** Longitudinal scan. Note spindle-shaped mass (M) which appears to be "splitting" the rectus muscle (arrow).

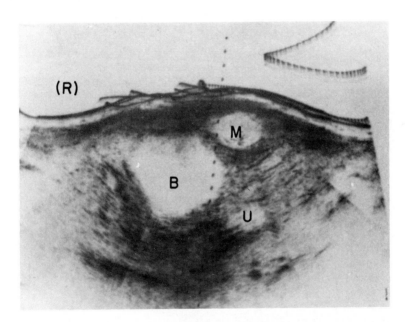

**Fig. 7-26.** Transverse scan. The mass (M) is anterior and to the left of the bladder (B).

DISCUSSION

To orient yourself to the longitudinal section, first identify the urinary bladder (Fig. 7-25, B). Anterior and cephalad to the bladder is a relatively sonolucent mass (M). Note that the mass is very superficial and seems to split the rectus muscle (arrow). Faint echo activity is noted within the mass. On the transverse section (Fig. 7-26), the bladder (B) is noted. The sonolucent mass (M) is anterior and slightly to the left.

FOLLOW UP

At surgery, a rectus sheath hematoma was found.

COMMENT

Five similar cases were recently reported by Kaftori and associates.[2] These authors have described rectus sheath hematomas as spindle-shaped on longitudinal scan and ovoid on transverse sections, a description that corresponds well with our experience.

## Case

OV is a 54-year-old female who presented with recently increasing abdominal girth. She was referred by her clinician, who wanted to know if she had ascites or an abdominal mass. Below are longitudinal and transverse scans (Fig. 7-27 and 7-28). What do you think?

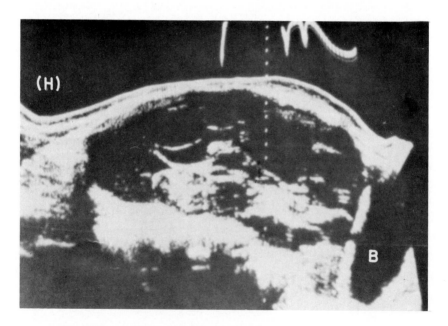

**Fig. 7-27.**   Supine longitudinal scan. The bladder (B) is labeled.

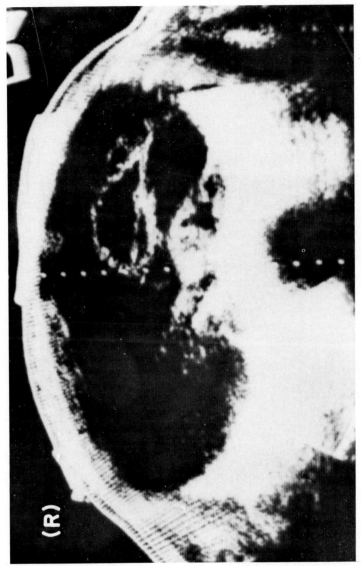

**Fig. 7-28.** Transverse scan at 4 cm above the umbilicus.

187

DISCUSSION

The transverse section (Fig.7-29A) revealed a large sonolucent mass within which there were recognizable structures (arrows). The borders of the mass appeared to be sharply defined. Compare this case to Fig. 7-29B below. Ascitic fluid (F) can be identified around the root of the mesentery.

The longitudinal scan (Fig. 7-30A) again reveals a sonolucent mass with multiple septa (arrows). Compare Fig.7-30A to the longitudinal scans in a patient with ascites (Fig. 7-30B, 7-30C). Ascitic fluid (F) is noted over the bladder, adjacent to the liver, and outlines bowel loops (arrows).

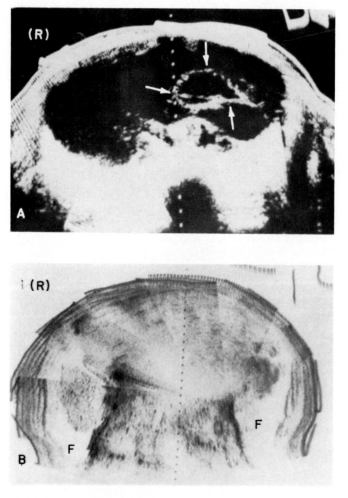

**Fig. 7-29.** (A) Transverse scan. Note septa (arrows). (B) Transverse scan. Ascitic fluid (F) is seen around the root of the mesentery.

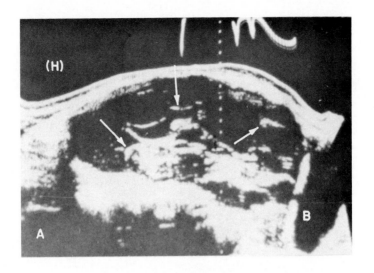

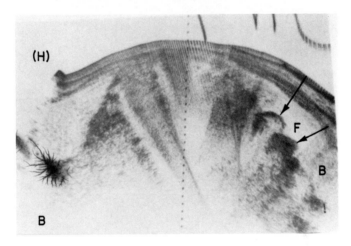

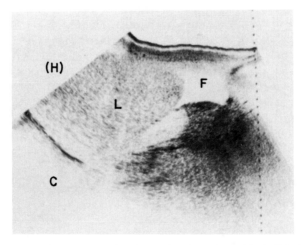

**Fig. 7-30.** Supine longitudinal scans. (A) Septa are present (arrows). (B) Ascitic fluid (F) is present and outlines bowel loops. (C) Note ascitic fluid (F) at tip of liver (L).

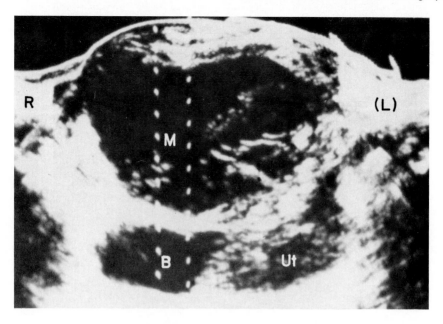

**Fig. 7-31.** Transverse scan. The relationship of the mass (M) to the bladder (B), uterus (Ut) can be appreciated.

FOLLOW UP

At surgery, a large serous cystadenocarcinoma of the ovary was found.

COMMENTS

When the suspicion of a mass arising from the pelvis is raised,it behooves the sonographer to perform a complete pelvic sonogram. Below is a transverse section of the pelvis in the patient introduced on p. 186 (Fig. 7-31). The bladder (B) is pushed to the right, while the uterus (Ut) is displaced to the left. The pelvic origin of the mass becomes more obvious. It is also of value, when a pelvic mass is identified, to check the kidneys for hydronephrosis secondary to obstruction of the ureters by the mass.

Aside from ovarian cysts, there are other masses that arise from the pelvis and extend up into the abdomen, such as uterine neoplasms, the pregnant uterus, hydatidiform moles, and so on. On occasion, particularly in males, a dilated urinary bladder may extend well up into the abdomen.

### Case

PO is a 60-year-old male admitted with abdominal pain. The first imaging procedure performed during this admission was a gallbladder sonogram. How much pathology can you identify on the representative longitudinal and transverse scans below (Fig. 7-32, 7-33, 7-34)?

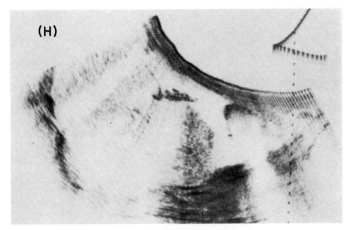

**Fig. 7-32.** Supine longitudinal scan.

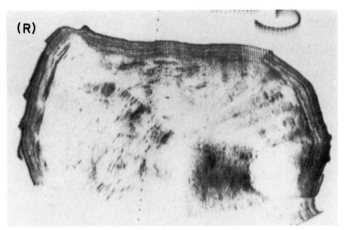

**Fig. 7-33.** Transverse scan at xyphoid −5 cm.

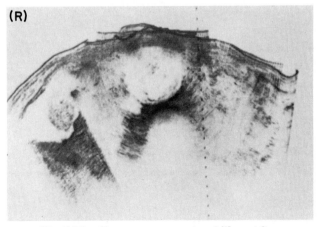

**Fig. 7-34.** Transverse scan at umbilicus +2 cm.

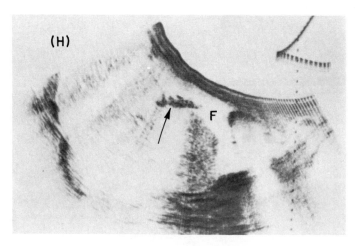

**Fig. 7-35.** Longitudinal scan. Gallstones (arrow) and ascitic fluid (F) are present.

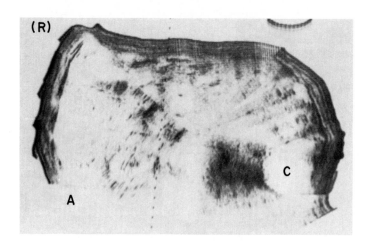

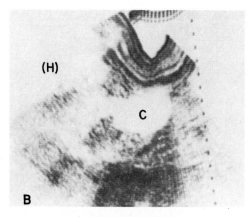

**Fig. 7-36.** (A) Transverse scan. There is a left renal cyst (C). (B) Prone longitudinal scan of the left kidney showing left renal cyst.

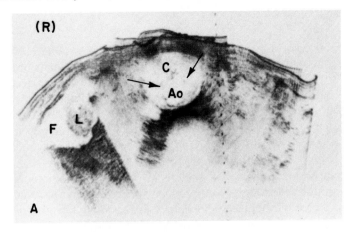

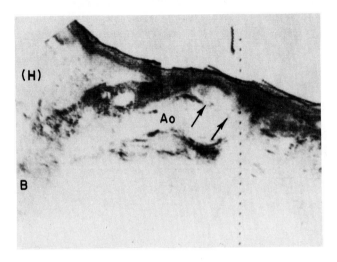

**Fig. 7-37.** (A) Transverse scan. There is an abdominal aortic aneurysm associated with a circumferential clot (C). Ascitic fluid (F) is again noted around the tip of the liver (L). (B) Supine longitudinal scan again showing aneurysm and clot (arrows).

DISCUSSION

Fig. 7-35 reveals the presence of gallstones (arrow) and ascites (F).

In the transverse scan (Fig. 7-36A) a left renal cyst (C) is identified and is confirmed by a prone longitudinal scan of the left kidney (Fig. 7-36B).

Finally, the transverse scan at 11 cm from the xyphoid (Fig. 7-37A) again reveals ascitic fluid (F) around the liver. In addition, an abdominal aortic aneurysm with intramural thrombus (arrows) is noted and confirmed on a longitudinal scan (Fig. 7-37B).

## SUMMARY

Ultrasound provides an excellent modality for the evaluation of abdominal aortic aneurysms. Appropriate longitudinal and transverse scans not only delineate the size of the aneurysm, but also reveal the presence of hematoma within the wall of the aneurysm. Retroperitoneal masses, such as lymphomas, may also be detected by ultrasound. Since these lesions may be relatively sonolucent, one must be certain that the mass is separate from aorta. Abdominal sonography also provides a noninvasive means of following the response of such masses to treatment.

Superficial abdominal masses, such as abscesses and hematomas, present as relatively sonolucent lesions. The rectus sheath hematoma localized low in the abdomen has a characteristic spindle-shaped appearance. Minimal ascites may be detected by means of ultrasonic evaluation of the abdomen. The fluid is usually located around the liver, the root of the mesentery, and over the urinary bladder.

Finally, abdominal masses that arise from the pelvis, such as ovarian cysts and fibroids, can be effectively evaluated by sonography. Complete evaluation of the pelvis in such cases will frequently reveal the orgins of the masses.

## REFERENCES

1. Kaftori JK, Rosenberger A, Pollack S, et al: Rectus heath hematoma: Ultrasonographic diagnosis. Am J Roentgenol 128:283–285, 1977
2. Steinberg I, Stein HL: Arteriosclerotic abdominal aneurysms. JAMA 195:1025–1029, 1966

# Index

a
b
c
d
e
f
9 g
0 h
1 i
8 2 j